CONTENTS

FOREWORD

The modern approach to diabetes is a positive one: we are now concerned with helping those with diabetes to keep fit and healthy. This splendid book is written in a clear and straightforward style by a Physician devoted to helping those with diabetes to help themselves. It contains much more than its title implies. It explains the role of sport and activity in the life of those with diabetes, how to avoid the risks of excessive exercise and how to enjoy the fruits of keeping fit.

The modern diabetic must control and manage his own health and future. The more he understands the nature of diabetes and how to control it, the better able he will be to sustain and maintain good health.

I commend this book with warmth and enthusiasm. Nobody with diabetes can fail to benefit from its perusal.

Arnold Bloom, M.D., F.R.C.P.
Consultant Physician

INTRODUCTION

My aim in this book is to provide the necessary information and advice for those who have insulin-treated diabetes who wish to take part in active sports and pastimes. I will try to illustrate various points with information based on my own and my patients' experience of diabetes and sport, but it is important to remember that each person is different and needs individual attention. What works for one, say with regard to the amount of extra carbohydrate taken before and after a game of squash, aerobics class or swimming session, may not work for another. The best plan for the individual can only be determined by trial and error, but if this is based on the previous experience of others then the errors should be fewer.

The advice and information in this book are not a substitute for a one-to-one discussion with the doctor, dietician or diabetic support nurse at the clinic. However, I am sure you will agree that these people are always very busy and if you can get some information from a book like this beforehand then it will be helpful in your discussions.

During the first part of this book I will describe how the metabolism of the body responds to exercise and particularly how the muscles obtain their extra fuel requirements. Of course, different sports and pastimes will vary in terms of the amount of energy expended; a hectic game of squash will make more demands on the body than a gentle stroll through the country-side. I will, therefore, outline the energy requirements for the different sports to enable you to plan your insulin injections and carbohydrate intake accordingly.

A large section of the book is devoted to the avoidance of

diabetic problems occurring when taking part in active sports. Important considerations here involve learning more about 'hypos' and their cause, the importance of measuring blood glucose levels and caring for the feet. Unfortunately, there are some sports that are unsuitable for the person with diabetes but, hopefully, when the reasons have been explained, you will agree and not be too disappointed that certain activities are best avoided. It is preferable to concentrate on those sports which can be performed safely and well. Sometimes there is a difference of opinion among doctors and diabetic people about which activities are suitable and how best to cope in terms of carbohydrate intake or insulin administration. I present my own views which I believe represent a fairly broad concensus.

In the past I have been involved as medical officer at summer camps, organised by the British Diabetic Association (B.D.A.). Looking after perhaps twenty very active diabetic teenagers for 2 weeks every year certainly makes one aware of the problems encountered and provides experience of how to solve them. The camps help the young to cope with the condition and also provide excellent holidays. I attach a great deal of importance to these camps and have devoted a chapter of this book to them. I have given the address of the B.D.A. on page 111 so that you will be able to get in touch and perhaps go on one of the camps.

I intend this book to highlight the advantages of incorporating sport and exercise into your daily programme as an aid to better control. Exercise has always been an important factor in the treatment of diabetes, together with insulin and diet, and can have profound effects on diabetic control in terms of blood glucose levels and insulin requirements. In addition, exercise and sport can have other beneficial effects, and I will describe these in some detail. I will have to be negative occasionally and point out that some people with diabetes perhaps ought not to take part in sport because of medical problems but often some form of exercise is still possible.

Some of my diabetic patients have told me in detail how they handle their diabetes when they take part in different sports. I have included this information so that you can benefit from their experience and can compare their diet and insulin adjustments with your own. They certainly do not let diabetes interfere with either their enjoyment of or ability at sport.

Young people taking insulin can take up fairly active sport from the outset so long as they pay attention to their diet and insulin. Older people on insulin, the same as older non-diabetics, are less physically adaptable and would have difficulties. This can be overcome to a certain extent by a gradual introduction to physical activity. However, older people who have had diabetes for many years may have other problems which need to be taken into account before starting to exercise, and I have included a chapter directed specifically at them.

A further objective of this book is to provide information which will be of value for those who come in contact with diabetic people during sporting activities, such as school teachers, youth leaders (for instance scouts and guides leaders, organisers of youth clubs, etc.), parents and sporting colleagues. For this reason, before discussing sport-related diabetic problems I will provide some background details of the nature of diabetes.

I hope you will find the book both enjoyable and informative and that it encourages you to take part in sport. It is my experience that people with diabetes prefer to know the facts and are far happier if they are aware of what to expect and how to avoid problems. This book is written in that spirit and aims to encourage rather than deter.

1

WHAT IS INSULIN DEPENDENT DIABETES?

This chapter should provide useful revision for the person taking insulin and information for those who come into contact with diabetic people during sporting activities. I am referring to schoolteachers who may be supervising sports sessions with a class which might include someone with diabetes, leaders in scout and guide packs, boys' brigades, cadets' organisations and youth clubs. Coaches at sports centres and supervisors at swimming baths should have some knowledge of diabetes, too.

Diabetes is a common disorder and is caused by a deficiency of insulin. Insulin is a hormone produced in specialised areas of the pancreas gland which lies at the back of the upper part of the abdomen. In 1921 Banting and Best extracted insulin from these specialised areas of the pancreas (pancreatic islets) which only comprise about 1g of tissue (the pancreas weighs approximately 50–75g in all). These researchers, working in Canada, showed that their pancreatic extract was capable of lowering the blood glucose in animals which had been made diabetic by the removal of the pancreas. Within a year of their discovery insulin was made available for the treatment of patients. Today very pure insulin is made from beef and pig pancreas and recently human insulin has become available which is made in bacteria by genetic engineering.

Insulin is a very important hormone in the body and its presence is necessary for life. The outlook, therefore, for young people with diabetes prior to the discovery of insulin was bleak. Today, those who need insulin treatment can live a normal life and can take part in most activities which involve physical exercise.

EFFECTS OF INSULIN ON THE BODY

Perhaps the best known effect of insulin is that of lowering the blood glucose level. If insulin production is deficient, then glucose entering the bloodstream after digestion of carbohydrate foods (such as bread, pastry, fruit, potatoes, chocolate) cannot be utilised by the body and therefore builds up in the blood. Glucose is an important fuel substance and failure to utilise it properly, due to lack of insulin, produces weakness and wasting. As well as not metabolising blood glucose derived from food, the body produces excess glucose in the liver during insulin deficiency. This process, called gluconeogenesis, pushes the blood glucose even higher.

Above a certain level (>10 mmol/l) glucose which is normally reabsorbed by the kidney spills out in the urine. This is called glycosuria. The presence of glucose in the urine also increases the amount of water and salt loss from the kidney. If this is severe, then dehydration occurs which, in some cases, can lead to shock. The loss of salt and fluid from the body reflexly stimulates thirst and these two factors, thirst and passing large amounts of urine (polyuria), together with weight loss and weakness, constitute the main symptoms of uncontrolled diabetes.

Insulin is important for the utilisation of blood glucose by the body and for controlling the production of glucose by the liver. In addition, insulin has important actions on the metabolism of other body fuels, particularly fat. In insulin deficiency the storage form of fat (triglyceride) is broken down and fatty acids are released into the blood stream. These substances, like blood glucose, are important body fuels and are further broken down, thereby yielding energy. The breakdown products of fatty acids are known as ketones. These substances are normally metabolised by the body but this depends on adequate insulin and glucose metabolism. So, in uncontrolled diabetes ketones accumulate in the blood and make the blood very acidic. Ketones also contribute to the loss of water and salts through the kidney.

The person who develops insulin dependent diabetes can become very sick, because of the marked effects of insulin deficiency on the body's metabolism, and in the beginning may need to be admitted to hospital for emergency treatment. However, once the initial metabolic disturbance is corrected,

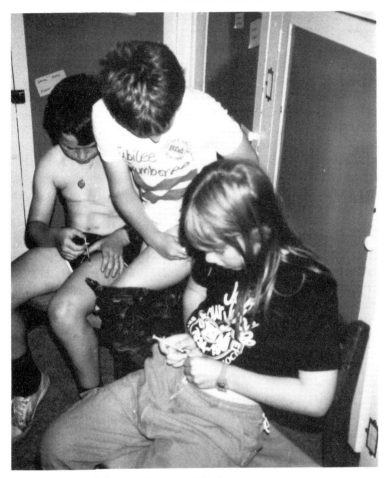

Injection time at a B.D.A. summer camp.

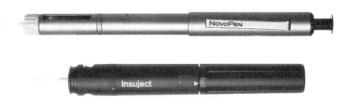

Pen injection devices.

often with the aid of a drip feed to restore body fluid and, of course, with insulin, the symptoms rapidly disappear and improvement is dramatic.

Insulin has to be given by injection and although the idea of having to inject insulin is daunting at first, most people manage without much difficulty, especially with the help of the new, very fine disposable needles and syringes. These cause very little discomfort when insulin is injected under the skin (subcutaneously). Insulin can be injected into several different sites (see pages 35–40), including the thighs and arms, but the abdomen is probably best. Care should be taken to vary the injection site, as continued injection into the same site can produce damage to the tissues underneath the skin.

Most people with diabetes inject insulin at least twice a day and sometimes more often, especially with the recent introduction of pen injection devices which make insulin injections much more convenient. Newly diagnosed diabetic people can often manage with one injection a day, but it is probably best to start on two injections from the onset as later on it may be difficult to persuade someone to increase the number of injections when this becomes necessary.

TYPES OF INSULIN

There are two main types of insulin, commonly known as clear and cloudy. The clear form is soluble insulin which, when injected under the skin, has a quick onset of action in lowering the blood glucose, but its period of action is relatively short. Cloudy insulin, on the other hand, is insulin either in the form of a suspension of insulin crystals or mixed with a substance, such as protamine, and produces a prolonged effect on blood glucose when injected under the skin, but with a slower onset of action. Examples of quick acting insulin are Actrapid, Velosulin, Neusulin, Humulin S, and intermediate acting insulin Monotard, Insulatard, Humulin Zn, Neuphane.

Most people with diabetes use a mixture of these short (clear) and longer acting insulins (cloudy), usually before breakfast and before the evening meal. This method produces four main peaks of insulin action. Other people use a single injection of a long lasting cloudy insulin at bedtime to provide a background level of insulin which is necessary for normal body metabolism, and before each meal use a quick acting insulin to provide the additional insulin needed to cover the meal. This system is much easier if the pen-injection devices are used.

BALANCE OF CARBOHYDRATE AND INSULIN

The injections of insulin need to be balanced by a regular intake of carbohydrate foods, avoiding those high in refined sugar, such as jams, marmalades, chocolate and cakes. The person with diabetes is seen by a diet expert (dietician) who makes an assessment of the total number of calories required daily. Obviously, this will vary from individual to individual, depending on age and activities. A balanced diet containing carbohydrate, fat and protein is then worked out to give the total amount of calories or fuel value needed for the day.

Until relatively recently the amount of carbohydrate in the diabetic diet was restricted, as it was thought that it was important for proper diabetic control. This is not the case and today people with diabetes will take up to 50 per cent of their total daily calories as carbohydrate, with the emphasis on foods high in fibre. The amount of animal fat in the diet is reduced. This dietary advice is in keeping with the so-called 'prudent diet' which is advocated for the population as a whole.

Approximately equal amounts of carbohydrate are eaten at each particular meal or snack. For instance, breakfast may consist of 40g carbohydrate; the mid-morning snack, 10g; lunch, 40g; tea, 10g; dinner, 50g; and the bedtime snack, 10g. To make it easier to take the same amount of carbohydrate at every breakfast, or other meal, a system of 10g carbohydrate exchanges has evolved so that although the total amount of breakfast carbohydrate is always 40g this can be made up by different foodstuffs. For instance, 5 tablespoons of cornflakes (10g) plus 2 thin slices of bread from a small loaf (20g) plus 1 large orange (10g) would make a total of 40g carbohydrate. Alternatively, 6 tablespoons of rice crispies (10g) plus 1 medium thick slice of bread from a large loaf (20g) plus a small carton of plain yoghurt (10g) would make a total of 40g. Similar principles are applied to other meals and snacks. For good diabetic control amounts of carbohydrate should be constant for a particular meal; ideally the timings of meals should be the same each day, and the injection timings should also be constant, i.e. 20–30 minutes prior to breakfast and the evening meal.

If the basal insulin requirement is separated from the insulin needed to cover meals by using a long acting insulin once a day, plus quick acting insulin before main meals, it is possible to be much more flexible in terms of meal times. People on twice-a-day mixtures of quick and longer acting insulin also have more flexibility in the timing of their evening meal if they 'split' the evening injection and have the quick acting insulin before the meal, whenever it is taken, and have the longer acting insulin before bedtime.

The balance between the insulin injected and the carbohydrate eaten is critical for maintaining a normal level of blood glucose. In the non-diabetic the output of insulin from the pancreas gland is under sensitive control. If no food is taken, then the output of insulin is very low. Conversely, if food is eaten, then the pancreas will respond by releasing a spurt of insulin.

What about the person with diabetes who depends solely on insulin injections? The main point is that once the insulin injection is given under the skin, then it will be absorbed into the blood stream at a rate determined by the particular sort of insulin. The level of blood glucose will not influence the absorption of this administered insulin. So, if the blood glucose is falling in the non-diabetic, normal insulin release from the pancreas will be 'switched off', but the injected insulin will continue to be absorbed. The major implication of this is the possible development of an abnormally low blood glucose, which is known as hypoglycaemia.

HYPOGLYCAEMIA

Hypoglycaemia has profound effects because the brain depends solely on blood glucose for its fuel supply in the short term, so that if the blood glucose is low the brain is starved of fuel for its metabolism and therefore does not function properly. The symptoms and signs of hypoglycaemia (a 'hypo') are fully described in Chapter 3 and it is important that everyone who has contact with diabetic people should be familiar with these symptoms. It is obviously advisable not only to be able to recognise hypoglycaemia but also to be able to administer first aid.

It is best to prevent hypoglycaemia, which is more likely to occur at certain times and under certain circumstances. If meals are missed or taken late, then there is a high risk of hypogly-caemia. So, a relatively simple measure in its prevention is to ensure that diabetic people do not miss and are not late for meals. Snacks taken between the main meals are equally important in this regard.

Exercise and sport can cause hypoglycaemia. In general, exercise will lower blood glucose in the person with diabetes and increase the likelihood of hypoglycaemia unless adequate precautions are taken. Chapter 3 discusses how to avoid problems occurring during physical activity. A point to remember is that you should be sympathetic towards the diabetic in terms of eating at fairly fixed times. This may mean eating a snack at a time when normally it would be against school rules.

Fortunately, problems resulting from the rapid development of a high blood glucose and subsequent acidosis, shock and coma are rare in diabetics and, hopefully, people at whom this chapter is aimed will not have to deal with the situation. However, it is worth knowing the circumstances in which it can arise.

KETOACIDOSIS

In my experience most cases involving the development of severe uncontrolled diabetes (known as diabetic keto-acidosis) in the established diabetic result from infections, such as gastroenteritis and chest infections. Any infection is a stressful event for the body and it responds by releasing various hormones which have the opposite effects on blood glucose to insulin. The body, therefore, becomes resistant to insulin and in the diabetic this causes the blood glucose to rise if the dose of administered insulin is not increased. If the blood glucose does rise, then the symptoms will be those of the person developing diabetes for the first time, which I described earlier. In such a situation it is advisable to get medical advice quickly and the nearest hospital casualty department is the safest answer. However, most diabetics cope very well with minor stresses, such as infections, and part of the education of the diabetic is devoted to ensuring an understanding and knowledge of how to react to these situations. Briefly, at times of illness the blood glucose should be monitored very carefully, at least four times during the day (see pages 33–5 for details of blood glucose measurements). A mistake often made is not to continue insulin injections because the appetite has been affected. The insulin dose may actually need to be increased, depending on the blood glucose measurements. People with diabetes are taught how to do this and additional injections of quick acting insulin may also be required. If the appetite is affected, then it is important to continue to take some carbohydrate. In this situation glucose-containing fluids are very useful and should be used to supply the relevant amount of carbohydrate. If vomiting occurs, then it is best to get medical help. This is not a case which the local doctor can deal with, so hospital is best.

In an attempt to improve communication between young diabetics and their parents and teachers at school the B.D.A. has developed a 'School Pack'. The information, which is printed on plastic cards, is easily assimilated, and provides advice to parents and schools, including suggestions for discussion with the headmaster, etc. I am sure that this B.D.A. publication will go a long way towards increasing teachers' awareness of the problems faced by young insulin dependent diabetics at school. The suggestions for discussion with head teachers, especially, provide a strong basis for meaningful interviews with parents. I

I AM A DIABETIC

NAME _____

ADDRESS _____

_____ Tel. No. _____

- IF I am unconscious or behaving abnormally, I may be having a reaction associated with diabetes or its treatment.
- IF I can swallow, give me sugar or a sweet drink. (There should be sugar or glucose tablets on my person).
- IF I do not recover promptly, call a doctor, or send me to hospital.
- IF I am unconscious or cannot swallow, do not attempt to give me anything by mouth, but call a doctor or send me to hospital immediately.

U-100 INSULIN DOSE CARD

USUAL HOSPITAL/
CLINIC _____
_____ Tel. No. _____

TIME	TYPE(S) OF INSULIN	UNIT DOSE
MORNING		
EVENING		

B·D **Better Diabetes Care**

Information card for the person on insulin to carry, with details of first-aid measures for a 'hypo'.

also feel that some of these points are invaluable for other people, such as scout and youth club leaders. The information for schools, then, covers some background information about insulin dependent diabetes, problems with diabetes and important points for the diabetic at school. The pack also contains information about school outings, trips and expeditions. A record card gives important information about parents' phone numbers and addresses, the hospital address, dosage of insulin and details of diet.

2

THE BODY'S RESPONSE TO EXERCISE

After vigorous activity, such as a football match or a game of squash, most players experience an immense sense of well being and pleasure. These sensations are felt at a conscious level by physically fit people after sport. However, for the non-fit the conscious sensations may not be at all pleasant, and aching muscles and shortness of breath may be experienced. These feelings actually tell very little of the incredibly complicated series of reactions going on at a subconscious level which enables the body to cope with the additional exertion. Just think of the fine controls necessary so that working muscle fibres can perform at a greatly increased tempo, as the body moves from the resting state to vigorous exercise.

The metabolic pathways in the body are arranged so that the internal composition of the body cells, the body water surrounding the cells and the circulating blood do not change significantly. Even small changes can be damaging, so the body has evolved a complex system to maintain the necessary balance of these substances. As previously discussed, the main disturbances in body metabolism for the person with diabetes are hypoglycaemia and ketoacidosis. When the blood glucose level falls below the usual precisely maintained normal level, the brain, which in the short term is entirely dependent on glucose, cannot function correctly. In ketoacidosis the metabolism of blood glucose is greatly reduced and the body switches over to the breakdown of body fat as an alternative source of fuel. The fuel forms of fat are called fatty acids, and when these substances are broken down in the body cells to produce energy waste products called ketone bodies are formed. These substances can be used by the body but, if insulin secretion is deficient, they accumulate making the blood very acid. These metabolic disturbances which occur in diabetics are serious and distressing but can be avoided by careful control and management. Major adjustments take place in the body's metabolism during exercise and the conditions of hypoglycaemia, and occasionally ketoacidosis, can occur with increased frequency if proper preventative measures are not taken.

CHANGES TO BODY METABOLISM

What are the changes that take place in the metabolism of the body during exercise? Just like a car engine which uses more petrol at higher speeds, the body's engine, the muscles, require more fuel during exercise – the more vigorous the exercise, the more fuel is needed. For muscles to function normally during exercise an increase in the delivery of fuels to the contracting muscles is necessary. In fact, fuel requirements may increase twenty times after only a few seconds of vigorous exercise. When more fuel is burned in working muscles more waste products are produced. These substances need to be got rid of quickly and efficiently because, if they accumulate, they rapidly reduce the capacity of the muscle cells for further work. An example of this, which most people are familiar with, is the aching pain in muscles after prolonged activity. This is thought to be due to accumulation of a waste product called lactic acid in the muscles. The body cells can only tolerate small changes from the normal degree of acidity and the accumulation of lactic acid, therefore, limits the amount of activity possible.

Other dramatic changes which need to be smoothly regulated by the body during exercise are the increased flow of oxygen to the working muscles, and the disposal of the heat generated by the increased metabolic activity in the muscles. After a few seconds of energetic exercise there will be changes in the heart, to the circulation and in the lungs. The heart rate speeds up, enabling an increased flow of blood to the muscles. This increased blood flow to the muscles has to be compensated by a reduction in the flow to other parts of the body, such as the skin and intestines which are not directly involved in exercise.

Of course, the response of the body to increased activity will depend on the nature of the exertion. This may be a short, sharp sprint to catch a fast disappearing bus, or a fairly gentle ramble through the countryside. In terms of training and lasting benefit the most useful types of exercise are brisk walking, cycling and swimming. These are fairly vigorous but can be maintained for a reasonable length of time.

It will be useful to consider the body's response to this sort of activity under various headings, starting with effects on the lungs, then the circulation, the disposal of waste products and, finally, fuel supply.

LUNGS

Oxygen is indispensable for metabolism and the body has evolved very efficient mechanisms for its transport and use. Air which contains about one fifth oxygen enters the lungs via the nose and mouth, passing along a series of tubes called bronchi; the lungs and the bony rib cage act as bellows during the act of breathing. The lungs lie in the space formed by the chest wall and below by the diaphragm, and are attached to the inside of this space. When the chest wall expands and the diaphragm descends during breathing the lungs expand and air is sucked in. The chest wall is moved by muscles which lie between the ribs, and the diaphragm itself contains muscle fibres. Not much muscular effort is needed in breathing out in the resting state, as the air is pushed out by the elastic recoil of the lungs. The lungs never empty completely and there is always a residual volume amounting to about a litre left in them even after the biggest breath out. The bellows effect enables a continuous transport of oxygen into the lungs and from there into the bloodstream, and continuous transport of carbon dioxide (a gas formed as a waste product during the body's metabolism) in the opposite direction.

The actual transfer of oxygen from the lungs to the blood and the transfer of carbon dioxide in the opposite direction take place in the lungs in microscopic air sacks known as alveoli. The alveoli are directly adjacent to small blood vessels called capillaries, which are only one cell thick. As the blood passes through the capillaries, oxygen diffuses across the wall of the capillary into the blood. This occurs because oxygen in the lungs is at a higher concentration than in the blood. Carbon dioxide diffuses in the opposite direction, as its concentration in the blood is higher than in the lungs. This process has to be very fast and efficient because during exercise the red cells of the blood, which carry the oxygen, pass through the capillary in less than a quarter of a second.

The amount of carbon dioxide is generally kept at a fairly constant concentration in the body because of the important effects it has on the acidity of the blood and the control of blood flow to the brain. If the amount of carbon dioxide in the blood rises, for any reason, the body reacts by stimulating breathing, so that more carbon dioxide is removed by the lungs and body levels can return to normal.

Exercise has, therefore, a marked effect on breathing because of the increased amounts of oxygen required, and the need to rid the body of the additional carbon dioxide formed. This can be seen when considering the actual volumes of air transferred during breathing. At rest, about 10 litres of air per minute are inhaled, by the breathing motion of the chest wall and diaphragm, into the lungs. During a brisk walk the amount of air taken in and out rises about six times to 60 litres each minute. So the lungs have a high reserve and, in the young fit person, this is generally more than enough to ensure adequate oxygen supply during exercise.

HEART AND CIRCULATION

Once the oxygen has entered the bloodstream through the lungs it is carried around the body by the red blood cells. These cells contain a substance called haemoglobin which is an iron-containing protein. Haemoglobin is able to bind and carry oxygen with remarkable efficiency; the haemoglobin in just one red blood cell is capable of carrying millions of oxygen molecules. Carbon dioxide is also carried in a similar manner by the red cells. The amount of oxygen which reaches the muscles depends on the ability of the blood to carry oxygen, the actual amount of blood flowing through the muscles and the ability of the muscle cells to extract the oxygen from the blood. It is these factors which ultimately limit the body's capacity to cope with vigorous exercise.

The freshly oxygenated blood from the lung capillaries re-enters the left side of the heart via a collecting chamber called the left atrium. A valve called the mitral valve, which only allows blood flow in one direction, separates the left atrium from the powerful pumping compartment of the heart which is called the left ventricle. Blood enters the left ventricle in a controlled way and is pumped by the contracting muscles of the heart from the ventricle into the aorta, the largest artery of the body. Another valve is present where the aorta joins the heart and this prevents blood flowing back into the heart. From the aorta the oxygenated blood is carried to all the organs and tissues of the body via a complex system of smaller blood vessels, eventually terminating in the capillary networks.

The pressure of blood in the arteries varies, depending on whether the left ventricle is contracting and therefore pumping blood into the aorta, or relaxing and allowing blood to enter from the left atrium and filling the ventricle before its next contraction. The peak pressure in the arteries at the time of contraction of the left ventricle is called systole, and the pressure when the left ventricle is relaxing is called diastole. Systolic pressure is about 120 mm of mercury under ordinary conditions, and about 80 mm during diastole. The difference between the systolic and diastolic pressure, the pulse, can be felt in arteries. Pressure is maintained in the arterial system when the heart is refilling, prior to its next contraction, because the walls of the arteries are elastic and there is some recoil of these elastic tissues during diastole. This property of the arteries is very important and enables pressure to be maintained between heart contractions, so that the blood supply to the various organs of the body is not interrupted.

As we have noted, during exercise the heart rate increases and this can be felt by an increase in the pulse. (You can feel your own pulse at the wrist in the radial artery.) While exercising, the heart can beat as fast as 200 beats per minute in children, and about 170 beats per minute in older people. Not only does the heart rate increase during exercise but also the amount of blood pumped out at each beat. This tends to increase the systolic blood pressure and helps to ensure that the increased blood flow to the muscles is maintained, without causing problems in the blood supply to other important organs. At rest each heart beat or contraction pumps about 70 mls of blood but on exercise this can rise to about 120 mls.

At rest, the muscles take about a quarter of the heart's output of blood but, when the muscles are involved in vigorous exercise, this can rise to about nine-tenths. The peak pressure in the arteries (systolic pressure) may then double but the diastolic pressure does not change very much. Hence, the pulse feels much more forceful when the body is exercising. The increase in pressure ensures that the blood flow to the brain is maintained during exercise, but some blood still has to be diverted from the kidneys and from the intestine. It is, therefore, unwise to exercise after a heavy meal.

Oxygen is taken up by the body tissues from capillaries which, you will remember, are only a single cell thick; carbon dioxide passes in the reverse direction. When the oxygen has passed to the tissues, the de-oxygenated blood travels back from the capillaries to the right side of the heart via the veins. There are a series of valve-like structures in veins which only allow the blood to flow one way, i.e. back to the heart. On this low pressure side of the circulation the pumping action is provided by the muscles surrounding the veins. Blood is then pumped through the lungs again by the right ventricle and so the process continues.

DISPOSAL OF WASTE PRODUCTS

Heat
The large increase in the metabolic activity of the muscles, which occurs during vigorous exercise, produces an increased amount of heat. To function efficiently and to avoid possible dangerous increases in body temperature, the body has developed ways of dispersing the excess heat. I am sure that you will have noticed during your sporting activities that you feel more comfortable in cool weather than in warmer weather – games such as soccer and rugby are played in winter for this reason. If the surroundings are cool then heat transfers more readily from the body surface to the air, particularly if there is a cool breeze blowing. In warmer surroundings, such as when you are taking part in a vigorous game of squash or badminton; then other mechanisms come into effect to increase heat loss. So that the body can balance the heat produced by the heat lost the blood flow to the skin is increased, allowing more heat to be lost directly to the air. You may have noticed after a game that your skin looks flushed and that you feel hot. This is because of the increased skin blood flow. Normally, less than two per cent of the total blood goes to the skin but it may increase to twenty per

cent after a period of heavy work. This means that the heart has to work much harder to supply the large increase in blood flow to the skin and also to keep up the supply to the muscles. So it is certainly a greater stress to the body to perform hard vigorous exercise in warm or hot surroundings than in a cooler environment. Sometimes in a really vigorous game of squash, for example, the need of the muscles for blood is so great that the flow to the skin is reduced and the regulation of the body temperature is sacrificed for a short time. Of course, it is only possible to keep up such a level of activity for a short period. After the game skin blood flow will increase rapidly and players who were pale and uncomfortable during the hard match become flushed and feel hot but generally more comfortable.

Another way the body loses heat is by sweating. As the sweat evaporates from the body, heat is removed. In very hard exercise sweating is increased dramatically, especially if performed in warm surroundings. The fluid lost from the body may be as much as 2 pints in an hour. Sweat not only contains water but also salt, so that if salt and water are not taken then this intense exercise soon becomes impossible. You will have seen marathon runners and long distance cyclists taking fluids during races. People with diabetes who are not well controlled are particularly prone to dehydration when taking part in vigorous sport on warm days.

Carbon dioxide
Another waste product of metabolism is carbon dioxide which is produced following the breakdown of glucose and fatty acids. Carbon dioxide diffuses out of the working muscle cells into the blood capillaries, as oxygen passes from the capillaries to the cells. It is carried in the blood returning to the heart and lungs by the veins. Once inside the lung capillaries carbon dioxide diffuses from the blood into the air spaces of the lung, leaving the body as air is breathed out. These movements of oxygen and carbon dioxide by the process of diffusion are possible because of the differences in their concentrations between different tissues. In working muscles where a lot of carbon dioxide is being produced the concentration will be higher than in the fresh blood arriving from the heart in the muscle capillaries. The flow of carbon dioxide is from the area of high concentration to the area of low concentration. On the other hand, the concentration of oxygen is higher in the blood entering the muscle

capillaries than it is in the muscle cells where it is being utilised. Therefore, oxygen moves in the opposite direction to carbon dioxide.

FUEL SUPPLY FOR WORKING MUSCLES

It will be easier to understand how diabetes affects the way the body copes with the additional energy demands of exercise and especially how this affects blood glucose, if we first consider what happens in the person without diabetes.

When muscles are resting they do not obtain much of their fuel from blood glucose. In fact in this situation when the muscles are not actively involved in contracting, most of their fuel supply is derived from the breakdown of fats. However, when muscles begin to contract at the start of exercise they receive most of their fuel from glucose stored in the muscle. The storage form of glucose is called glycogen. It is very important for the first 5–10 minutes of exercise. This store of energy continues to provide some fuel for the working muscles, but the glucose delivered to the muscles in the bloodstream becomes more important. The blood supply to working muscles is dramatically increased and is able to deliver fuel substances such as glucose more speedily. In fact, following the first 10 minutes or so of exercise, muscles take up glucose from the bloodstream at up to 40 times the rate at rest.

You will remember that in resting muscle blood glucose is relatively insignificant as a source of fuel. However, during exercise blood glucose provides approximately 40 per cent of the total energy requirements of the muscles. The rate at which glucose is used by the muscles increases as the muscles continue to exercise and reaches a peak at about 2 hours, after which there is a small fall. Along with the increasing use of blood glucose as a fuel during prolonged exercise muscles are also utilising fatty acids as fuel and, after about 4 hours of continuous exercise, the energy derived by muscle from fatty acids is approximately twice that from blood glucose (see Fig. 1).

Over a prolonged period of moderate exercise the fuel requirements of muscle are met initially from muscle glycogen, then predominantly from blood glucose and later from fatty acids. During very heavy exercise it seems that there is a more persistent dependence on the stores of muscle glycogen for

SHORT TERM EXERCISE

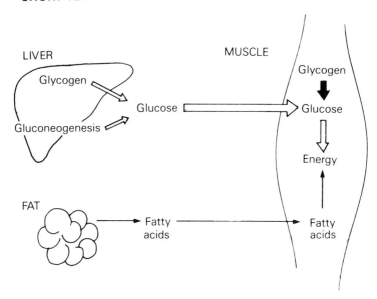

LONG TERM EXERCISE

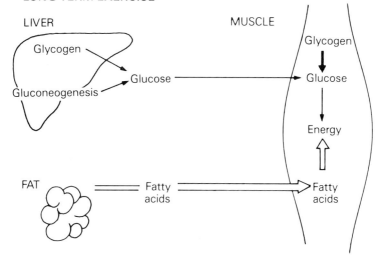

Fig. 1 After about 4 hours of continuous exercise, the energy derived by muscle from fatty acids is approximately twice that from blood glucose.

energy and the onset of fatigue appears to coincide with depletion of muscle glycogen.

We have seen that during exercise there is a dramatic increase in the uptake of blood glucose by the muscles to cope with the greater need for fuel. In the non-diabetic, however, the actual level of blood glucose changes very little. Even with prolonged exercise only a small fall of blood glucose is seen. A fall in blood glucose low enough to produce symptoms is very rare indeed in non-diabetics and is occasionally seen in people who have taken a diet very low in carbohydrate and in marathon runners.

During exercise the muscles utilise considerably more blood glucose and the actual blood glucose levels change very little. There must, therefore, be an increase in production of blood glucose. The liver is able to contribute to the level of blood glucose either by the process known as gluconeogenesis or by breakdown of glycogen, which is a storage form of glucose in the liver. The output of glucose by the liver may increase up to 5 times during short periods of exercise, depending on the intensity of the work performed. In the early period of sustained exercise the increased production of blood glucose by the liver comes mainly from the breakdown of glycogen. If exercise is more prolonged (over about 40 minutes), then the production of blood glucose in the liver by gluconeogenesis becomes more important. In fact the rate of liver production of blood glucose increases about three-fold when exercise is prolonged and the glycogen is gradually used up.

These changes in blood glucose output by the liver to compensate for the increased use of glucose as a fuel by the exercising muscles are brought about by the level of certain hormones in the blood during exercise. One of the most important hormones involved is obviously insulin. Levels of insulin fall during exercise, especially over long periods, and this probably results from the effects of the sympathetic nervous system. The fall in insulin causes an increase in the production of blood glucose in the liver by gluconeogenesis, a process which is usually inhibited by insulin. If exercise is severe or prolonged, other hormones including glucagon and adrenaline also contribute to the provision of blood glucose by the breakdown of glycogen and increased gluconeogenesis.

3

EXERCISE IN THE DIABETIC

In the young insulin-taking diabetic the body's response to exercise with respect to the lungs, heart and circulation and the disposal of waste products will be essentially the same as that of the non-diabetic. In the older person with diabetes, however, there may be changes in the way the body reacts and additional factors related to the diabetes itself may need to be taken into consideration. Chapter 8 deals specifically with the problems which may arise in the older diabetic.

The main difference in the body's response to exercise in the young person with diabetes, is in the regulation of blood glucose levels. As we have seen, in the non-diabetic insulin levels in the blood fall during exercise because insulin secretion is blocked. This enables the liver to produce much needed glucose to supply the working muscles with fuel by the break-down of liver glycogen and the process of gluconeogenesis. If we compare this situation with that in diabetes we note the difference in the amount of insulin in the bloodstream. In the diabetic the level of insulin does not fall but can actually rise. This is because the speed at which insulin gets into the blood from the injection site under the skin generally stays the same (or may increase). As a result, the normal process which the body follows to increase the amount of glucose available as muscle fuel is blocked, i.e., the breakdown of liver glycogen to give glucose and the production of new glucose in the liver by gluconeogenesis. Despite this the insulin in the blood allows the muscle cells to go on taking up glucose for fuel. This means that glucose will be used up but will not be replaced. The obvious result of the unbalanced production and use of blood glucose is that the blood level will be reduced and may fall sufficiently to give a 'hypo' (see Fig. 2).

Hypoglycaemia is the main diabetic problem for those on insulin taking part in sport. Sporting exercise to 'burn up' the blood glucose is no substitute for good diabetic control. Exercise can be dangerous in poorly controlled diabetes and may lead to an increase in blood glucose and the development of ketoacidosis, as I will describe in more detail later.

SYMPTOMS OF HYPOGLYCAEMIA

Before talking about the avoidance of 'hypos' during and after exercise, it is worth saying a little more about 'hypos' in general. It is obviously important that before tackling any form of exercise the person with diabetes should be aware of 'hypo' symptoms, how to avoid them and how to treat them.

The blood glucose stays within fairly narrow limits (about 3–7 mmol/l) in non-diabetics. In people with diabetes the blood glucose before treatment tends to be high because there is a deficiency of insulin. Insulin treatment returns the blood glucose towards the normal range and symptoms of diabetes, thirst, the passing of large quantities of urine and weight loss are rapidly corrected.

Unfortunately, as we all know, insulin treatment has to be given by injection which is a disadvantage. However, most people get over the initial problems and, now that disposable syringes are available, injections become almost as routine as brushing the teeth. An important problem with the injection is the lack of flexibility once the insulin has been injected. Normally the pancreas can adjust its release of insulin into the bloodstream depending on the level of the blood glucose. In particular, if no food is taken and so no glucose is being absorbed from the intestine into the blood, then insulin release from the pancreas will be reduced. Consider the situation in the insulin-taking person following an injection of insulin. Once the injection is given, then the absorption of insulin from the injection site cannot be regulated and, even if no food is taken, the insulin continues to be absorbed. As a result, the blood glucose may fall to a low level producing symptoms of hypoglycaemia. The number of 'hypos' can be greatly reduced by taking some simple common sense precautions. Firstly, all people with diabetes should be aware of the symptoms of a 'hypo'. There are many of

NON-DIABETIC

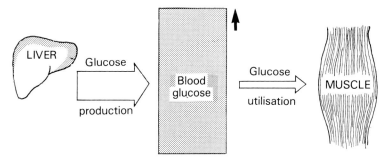

POORLY CONTROLLED DIABETES

ADEQUATELY CONTROLLED DIABETES

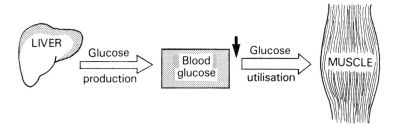

Fig. 2 The balance between glucose production and glucose utilisation in the non-diabetic, and in the poorly controlled and adequately controlled diabetic, during exercise.

these symptoms (see Fig. 3) and it is interesting that each individual very often has his or her own particular symptom or warning which is usually the same each time a 'hypo' occurs. In my patients the commonest warning symptoms tend to be a tingling of the lips or tongue, an intense hunger, and feeling hot and sweaty.

SYMPTOMS OF HYPOGLYCAEMIA (A 'HYPO')

Sweating
Feeling of intense hunger
Nervousness
Numbness   Due to the release of the
Pins and needles   stress hormone
Weakness   adrenaline from the
Heart palpitations   adrenal gland
Trembling

Slurring speech
Drowsiness
Confusion
Loss of memory   Due to inadequate
Irritability   supply of glucose to the
Headache   brain
Unsteadiness
Blurring of vision
Loss of consciousness
Convulsions

Fig. 3 Symptoms of hypoglycaemia.

Depending on the type of insulin used and when this is injected 'hypos' tend to be more likely to occur at particular times. A knowledge of this makes it possible to predict the time of greatest risk and to act accordingly. For instance, if an injection of soluble or short-acting insulin is given, say about 30 minutes before breakfast, then the maximum effective insulin action in lowering blood glucose will be 2 to 4 hours afterwards.

Therefore, it is possible to predict that the 'hypo' danger time will be before lunch. Knowing this it is easy to take preventative action which involves eating a snack (10–12g carbohydrate) midway through the morning and taking the midday meal on time.

For soluble insulin injected before an evening meal the 'hypo' danger time will be late evening and a 'hypo' at this time can be prevented by taking a bedtime snack. Most people on insulin in addition to taking short-acting soluble insulin in the morning and evening also take an intermediate-acting insulin. The 'hypo' danger times for these insulins are different from the short-acting soluble insulin, because their absorption is delayed from the injection site. Intermediate-acting insulin taken before breakfast will act strongly at around tea time. For this reason a mid-afternoon carbohydrate snack is important. An evening injection of intermediate-acting insulin will have its maximum effect in the early hours, which is another good reason for a bedtime snack. If 'hypos' are a problem at this time, then often they can be avoided by taking the intermediate-acting insulin at bedtime rather than before the evening meal.

Hypoglycaemic reactions are, to a large extent, avoided by having main meals on time and carbohydrate snacks between main meals to buffer the action of insulin at the times when it is strongest. In well controlled diabetes some hypoglycaemic symptoms may be felt just before meals and this is usually rapidly corrected by the meal.

It is important that at the first warning of a 'hypo' carbohydrate is taken in a form that will be absorbed rapidly into the bloodstream and will increase the blood glucose again. It will be obvious that wholemeal bread is not the right thing to take in such a situation, as its absorption will not be quick enough. Dextrosol tablets are probably the easiest and most convenient form of rapidly absorbable glucose. For people who drive a supply of Dextrosol should always be kept in the car. At home Lucozade, Pepsi or Coke are very useful.

One of the most frequent questions which I am asked by those on insulin is what will happen to them if they fall unconscious with a 'hypo' when they are on their own. Obviously, this is a very distressing thought but if the advice and guidelines I have just given are followed then it will be a very rare event; generally an individual will only experience 1 or 2 of these serious 'hypos'. The body responds to a 'hypo' by secreting hormones which tend to put up the blood glucose. One of these hormones called

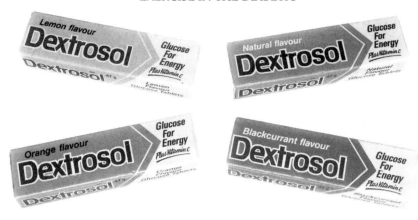

adrenaline tends to produce the first symptoms of the 'hypo'. Adrenaline and other hormones such as cortisol and glucagon are produced naturally by the body and they increase the production of glucose in the liver, so helping to restore the blood glucose to normal. This mechanism, together with the wearing off of the injected insulin, leads to recovery from unconsciousness.

It is of considerable importance for the family, workmates, schoolfriends and teachers of a diabetic person on insulin, to know about diabetes and the effects of a 'hypo'. Some people may occasionally become aggressive or confused during a 'hypo'. Speech may also be affected during a 'hypo' and it may not be possible to inform colleagues or school friends of the need for glucose. Another helpful measure is always to carry an information card. The card produced by the British Diabetic Association says simply 'If found ill, give two tablespoons of sugar in water'. Identification bracelets or necklaces are also very useful.

I have already said that in a serious 'hypo' the body by natural processes will restore the blood glucose to normal. However, it is obviously preferable if treatment is given in addition. The best treatment for this serious kind of 'hypo' is an injection of a concentrated glucose solution into a vein. This can only be performed by a doctor and so either an emergency call to the local doctor is necessary or a call for an ambulance to take the person to the nearest hospital with an accident and emergency

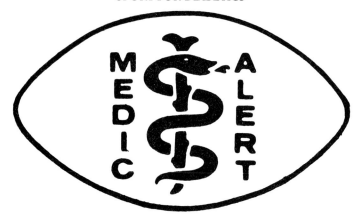

The emblem of an identification bracelet.

department. A technique that can often save these visits from the doctor or admissions to hospital is the injection of a hormone called glucagon. You will remember that this hormone, which like insulin is produced in the pancreas, raises blood glucose. Glucagon can be given by an injection into the muscles and so is easier to learn. More and more people with diabetes are keeping an ampoule of glucagon at home for emergency use by relatives who are taught how to give the injection. The response to glucagon takes about 5–10 minutes. When the person is roused sufficiently then glucose is also given by mouth. If glucagon is going to work in relieving a 'hypo' it does so within 10–15 minutes; if there has been no effect by this time, then a call to the doctor or hospital is necessary.

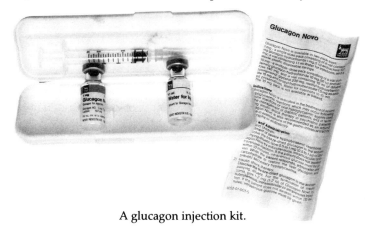

A glucagon injection kit.

HOME MONITORING OF BLOOD GLUCOSE

To achieve good diabetic control, which is essential for sport, it is important to be able to measure blood glucose levels. In recent years, simple techniques for blood glucose measurements which can be performed at home have been developed.

Testing urine for glucose is inconvenient and bears little relationship to the blood glucose level. This is because the level of blood glucose at which glucose appears in the urine varies markedly between different people and also from day to day in any one person. Above a blood glucose level of about 10 mmol/l the kidneys cannot reabsorb all the glucose passing through them and glucose spills over into the urine. This is called the renal (kidney) threshold for glucose. If good control is the aim then a blood glucose of over 10 mmol/l before a meal would not be satisfactory and so, assuming an average renal threshold, the person with well-controlled diabetes should have all negative tests for urine glucose. Then arises the problem, as many diabetics have expressed it to me, 'how negative is negative?' In other words, when the urine test is blue (that is, negative for glucose on Clinitest) it is impossible to know if this means a satisfactory blood glucose level or one that is too high, or if the danger of a 'hypo' is imminent.

For the diabetic person who wishes to take part in sport these problems are obviously even more important. Self-monitoring of blood glucose is an innovation which certainly allows more intelligent control of diabetes during sport and everyday life, and can give much more reassurance than urine testing. Quite young children are capable of self-monitoring and it is my experience, and that of others who have looked after children on B.D.A. holidays, that about 9 out of 10 children prefer self-monitoring of blood glucose to urine testing.

The equipment now available for blood glucose measurement enables testing to be performed more or less anywhere. The automatic finger pricking devices, which allow blood samples to be obtained from the finger without discomfort, have made self-monitoring acceptable to the great majority of people with diabetes. The three instruments for finger pricking with which I am personally familiar are the 'Autolet', the 'Autoclix' and the 'Autolance'. These machines are easy to use and painless and, as can be seen from the photographs (see page 34), are small and easily carried about. They also only cost a few pounds and are well worth the investment. The three machines can be obtained from the address shown on page 111.

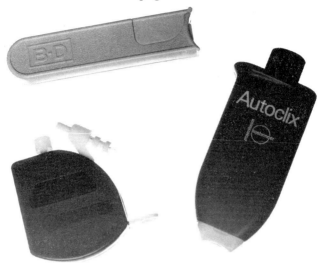

The 'Autolance' (top), 'Autolet' (bottom left) and 'Autoclix' (bottom right) finger pricking machines.

Once the sample of blood is obtained it is placed on a specially designed blood glucose testing strip for a set time. The blood is then wiped off and the colour of the strip changes depending on how much glucose is in the blood. The colour on the strip is matched against a colour chart. These testing strips only give accurate results if used correctly. It is most important that an adequate drop of blood is placed on the strip (not smeared on!) and that the timing is accurate (use the second hand of a watch, do not try to guess the time). Several blood testing strips are available with different colours. Find which is the easiest for you to use with the help of the clinic doctor or liaison nurse.

For those who have difficulty with reading the blood testing strips, small battery operated machines are available which have optical devices for reading the colour reaction on the strips. The three machines commonly in use for self-monitoring in the U.K. are the Glucochek, Hypocount and Glucometer. I have had experience with all three of these machines and find them very effective if used correctly. However, a possible danger with the machines is that they may always be believed to be right. The machines as well as the reagent strips, are only as good as the people using them. If the machines are used incorrectly, they will give invalid results. For this reason people should be thoroughly trained in their use. As an additional check the reagent strip can always be read in the usual way against the colour chart. The machines are portable and can be stowed with sports kit to allow a blood glucose test to be performed at a convenient time before and during sporting activity.

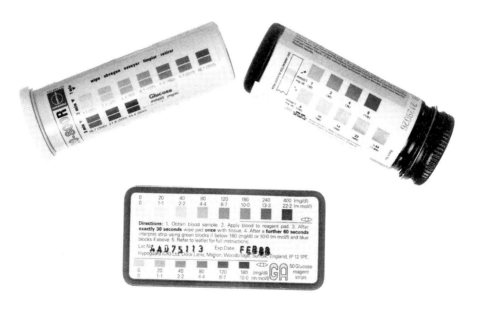

Different testing strips for home blood glucose monitoring.

INJECTION SITES AND INSULIN ABSORPTION

A potentially important mechanism contributing to the increased risk of a 'hypo' during sport is the possible effect of exercise on the absorption of insulin injected under the skin. If the speed at which insulin reaches the bloodstream from the injection site increases, this in turn increases the 'hypo' risk. More time will be spent on the problem later, but first of all some general aspects of insulin absorption from injection sites need to be considered.

The influence of the injection site on the absorption of insulin and diabetic balance has been apparent to people with diabetes and their doctors for many years. Fortunately, some factors involved in the variable absorption of insulin – the development of local changes in the fat under the skin (sometimes hard fatty lumps and sometimes marked loss of fat) at the injection site – have become less common due to the use of the newer 'mono component' or 'highly purified' insulins. These insulins are much purer than the older so-called 'dirty insulins'. However, it is still important to rotate the injection sites and to ensure that repeated injections at the same site are avoided (see Fig. 4). Some people with diabetes have difficulty injecting into their arms and, of course, if any bruises or skin changes do occur these will be visible for anyone wearing short sleeves. So, I do not recommend arms as injection sites.

The results of some recent research work involving the effect of various injection sites on insulin absorption are very interesting. Diabetic people volunteered for this study which was performed in America. All the volunteers had previously practised a very careful injection technique, with rotation of the injection sites. As a result, none of these people had any fatty lumps or other skin changes at the injection sites. On three different days the volunteer had an injection in either the arm, thigh or abdomen of a small amount of an experimental quick-acting soluble insulin. This experimental insulin had been made slightly radioactive, so that the amount of insulin under the skin could be measured with a Geiger counter. They also had ordinary cloudy insulin injected in the same area. After the insulin injections identical breakfasts were eaten.

The doctors carrying out these experiments took very great care to make sure that apart from different injection sites all other conditions for the experiments were the same on the three study days. The disappearance of the experimental radioactive insulin from under the skin was measured with a Geiger counter. The blood glucose concentrations of the volunteers were checked before and every quarter of an hour after the insulin injections and breakfast.

It was discovered that the area from which the radioactive soluble insulin was absorbed most quickly was the abdomen, followed by the arm; the slowest absorption was from the thigh. In fact, the differences were quite marked so that by 2 hours 15 minutes after the injection, 80 per cent more insulin had been

CHOOSING THE INJECTION SITE

THE MOST SUITABLE PLACES FOR INSULIN INJECTIONS ARE
GENERALLY THOSE AREAS OF THE BODY INDICATED BELOW:

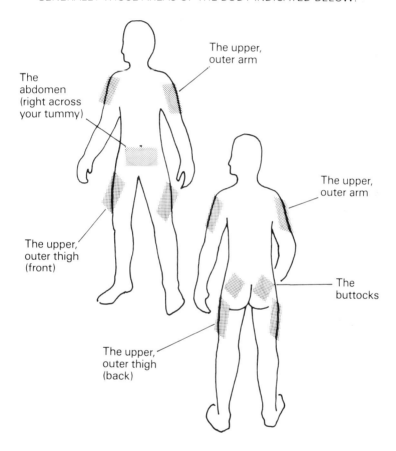

Fig. 4 Suitable sites for insulin injection.

absorbed from the abdomen compared with the leg. This was
found in all the volunteers studied. In turn, insulin absorption
from the arm was about 40 per cent more than from the leg but
about 30 per cent slower than absorption from the abdomen. It
is perhaps easier to appreciate these results by studying Fig. 5.

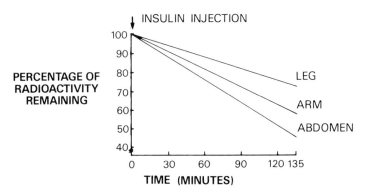

Fig. 5 Diagram showing the disappearance of radioactive insulin from injection sites in the abdomen, arm and leg. It is fastest from the abdomen, and then from the arm and from the leg.
(Redrawn from Koivisto and Felig, *Annals of Internal Medicine*, 1980, 92 (59–61))

As expected, the researchers found the changes in the absorption of insulin produced changes in the blood glucose measurements. The results were quite striking and blood glucose measurements in patients following the injection of insulin in the abdomen were much lower than when given in the arm or the leg (see Fig. 6). One explanation for the differences in insulin absorption, is that the blood supply to the fat under the skin of the abdomen is richer than that in the arm or leg.

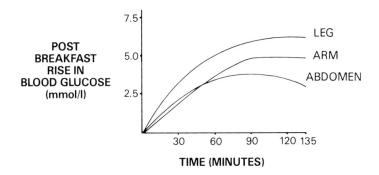

Fig. 6 Diagram showing the rise in blood glucose after breakfast, following the injection of insulin in different injection sites. The smallest rise in blood glucose occurs after an insulin injection in the abdomen.
(Koivisto and Felig, 1980)

Other important factors may affect the flow of blood in the small blood vessels around the injection site and so influence insulin absorption. For instance, blood flow can be affected by a hot bath. You will have noticed after a hot bath that your skin looks flushed. This is because there is more blood flowing through the skin blood vessels which dilate or get bigger in response to the warm conditions. A hot bath taken soon after an insulin injection may well affect the speed at which the insulin enters the blood stream. An increase in the rate of absorption of insulin can also occur on very hot days through a similar effect on skin blood flow.

A factor that indirectly affects skin blood flow which may not be so obvious is smoking. I would hope that any person with diabetes sufficiently interested to read this book will be concerned enough about health not to smoke. Apart from lung cancer, chronic bronchitis and premature disease of the arteries leading to heart attacks, strokes and gangrene of the legs, cigarette smoking may promote poor stabilisation of blood glucose control. The drug contained in cigarette smoke called nicotine can have quite dramatic effects on blood vessels, leading to a marked fall in the blood flow at the injection site. This has been shown by a group of diabetic research workers from Denmark. They found that, on average, diabetics who smoked seemed to need significantly more insulin than diabetics who were non-smokers. They performed scientific experiments on volunteers in which they tried to measure the effect of smoking on the absorption of insulin from the injection site. They injected radioactive insulin in the thighs of the volunteers. The rate at which the insulin was absorbed was then measured using a Geiger counter to count the amount of radioactive insulin left under the skin. The effect of smoking was quite dramatic. If the volunteers smoked just one cigarette, the rate at which the insulin was absorbed was reduced by half and this effect lasted for an hour. The implications for smokers are that the effect of nicotine on insulin absorption can cause unstable diabetes.

There are several known (and probably many unknown) factors which affect insulin absorption from the site of injection under the skin. It is important to take these into account when planning your own injections. Therefore, remember to rotate the site of the insulin injection to avoid producing fatty lumps. If you are unfortunate enough to have developed fatty lumps, avoid injecting into them. Since insulin absorption is different from one site to another, do not inject into the thigh one morning and into the arm the following morning. Try to be consistent. Because of these problems many of my patients only use their abdomen for injections, always making sure, of course, not to inject repeatedly into the same spot. You might think that you will run out of space but there is no likelihood of this happening; there are people who have given themselves insulin injections for over fifty years.

EFFECTS OF EXERCISE ON INSULIN ABSORPTION

Now that we have discussed some of the general factors affecting insulin absorption, we can look at the effects of exercise on insulin absorption.

A group of research workers in America set out to discover whether exercise (they chose in this case exercise on a fixed bicycle) affected the absorption of insulin injected under the skin in different sites of the body. First thing in the morning the volunteers were given identical breakfast meals and their insulin injections. The short-acting or clear soluble insulin was made radioactive so that it could be measured at the injection site using a Geiger counter. The volunteers were studied on different occasions after insulin injections into the arm, thigh and abdomen. Five minutes after the insulin injections the volunteers started to exercise and the radioactive insulin absorbed from the particular injection site was measured. Blood glucose measurements were also taken during the exercise, which lasted for an hour, and for several hours after the end of the exercise.

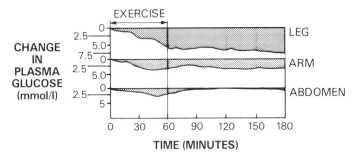

Fig. 7 Diagram showing the effects of insulin injected at different sites in reducing blood glucose following a period of exercise.

From these experiments the American researchers produced some interesting results which are very relevant to those of you who are keen on sport and exercise. It was discovered that the site where insulin was injected, prior to exercise, had an important effect on the speed at which insulin was absorbed into the bloodstream. Exercise considerably increased insulin absorption when insulin was injected into the thigh. During the hour's exercise 50 per cent more insulin was absorbed from the thigh compared with the amount absorbed when resting. The rate of insulin absorption was highest in the first 10–20 minutes of exercise, resulting in a bigger fall in blood glucose during the exercise period. Much larger falls in blood glucose were seen after the injection of insulin into the thigh, compared with arm and abdomen injections. The explanation for the increased absorption of insulin from the thigh during leg exercise is not fully understood but it may be related to the increased flow of blood to the leg because of the working leg muscles.

Some British diabetic investigators have also studied the effect of exercise on insulin absorption. In these experiments the investigators used volunteers who did not suffer from diabetes. These volunteers received an insulin injection into the thigh and then exercised on a fixed bicycle. Changes in the insulin levels in their blood were measured and compared with measurements from the same volunteers on other occasions when, instead of exercising, they rested in an armchair following the insulin injections. The dose of insulin given to these volunteers was, of course, small so as not to make them 'hypo'. The results of this research work are shown in Fig. 8. When the volunteers exercised after the insulin injection into the thigh, the amount of insulin in the bloodstream rose quite sharply, proving once again that the absorption of insulin into the leg increases when the leg is exercised.

It is important to point out here that another group of diabetic researchers did not find this effect of exercise on insulin absorption in their experiments. They did find that exercise lowered blood glucose but also that there was no increased disappearance of radioactive insulin from the injection site. Nor did they see any differences when insulin was injected into different sites. In these experiments the researchers did not ask the volunteer diabetics to start exercising until half an hour after the injection, whereas in the other studies exercise was started almost straight away after the injection. It could be that exercise

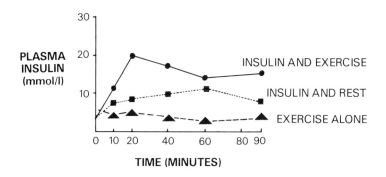

Fig. 8 The effect of exercise on the blood insulin concentration following an insulin injection into the thigh. Note that the insulin levels are higher after exercise than before exercise.
(Redrawn from Dandona et al, *British Medical Journal* (1978))

only affects the absorption of insulin if started immediately after the injection.

Studies which I have discussed so far have described the effects of exercise on the absorption of soluble quick-acting insulin. The effect of exercise on the absorption of intermediate- or long-acting insulins has not been studied in such detail. However, from the information available, it appears that after injection with the longer-acting insulins, there is an extended period of time in which the absorption can be affected by exercise.

CARBOHYDRATE INTAKE

The exercise which forms part of normal everyday life (such as walking, cycling or housework, etc.) for the person with diabetes is taken into account when the doctor and dietician discuss an individual's diet. Somebody who expends a lot of energy because of an active job will need more calories than someone who leads a more sedentary life. Another important factor which is taken into account is the person's weight and whether weight reduction is necessary.

Recently there has been a change in the dietary recommendations given to people with diabetes. Previously, advice on diet had been influenced to a certain extent by that given in pre-insulin days. Before insulin was introduced for the treatment of diabetes in the early 1920s the only treatment for diabetic people was severe carbohydrate restriction. After insulin became available the amount of carbohydrate included in the diet gradually increased. The carbohydrate allowance prescribed by Dr Lawrence for his diabetic patients on insulin in the 1920s and 1930s was very low, sometimes less than a 100g each day.

We know now that diabetic control can be just as effective with a higher carbohydrate intake, especially when the fibre content is high. The high carbohydrate, high fibre diet may also have additional benefits, for example, in lowering blood fats. This sort of diet has now been formally adopted by the British Diabetic Association. If you have not become familiar with the diet, then I can recommend a paperback book called *The Diabetic's Diet Book* by Dr Jim Mann and the dieticians in Oxford, which will give you all the information you need.

Exercise above the usual day-to-day routine is a special circumstance for the person with diabetes, because of the reasons I have already discussed. If this is to be enjoyed and 'hypos' prevented, then it is necessary to take additional carbohydrate to replace the glucose which exercise uses up. What type of extra carbohydrate to eat will obviously vary with the type of sport or exercise, particularly if it is relatively shortlived but strenuous, or less strenuous but more prolonged.

The muscular activity involved in sports, such as swimming, squash, running, ice skating, football, rugby and tennis, leads to the consumption of glucose at a very fast rate. For instance, a person swimming the butterfly stroke at a speed of approximately 50 yards a minute will consume in the region of 400 calories in half an hour. To give some idea of what this represents in terms of the increase in the body's energy expenditure, compare it with sitting still in a chair when the body uses in the region of 45 calories in half an hour. A list of the calories expended by various sports and activities is shown in Fig. 9. The values can only be approximate, however, as they depend on the skill attained at the particular sport and the effort put into it. If competition is involved then generally this leads to more effort and consequently more calorie consumption. The calories used will also depend on body weight. If a person is overweight then he or she will probably expend more energy.

If you know the calorie consumption of the activity it is possible to work out the approximate amount of extra carbohydrate which is required to cover the exercise and prevent a

LIGHT WORK (energy use 2.5-4.9 calories/minute)

Bowling
Walking slowly
Cycling (5 mph)

MODERATE WORK (energy use 5.0-7.4 calories/minute)

Golf	Badminton
Walking briskly	Table tennis
Ballroom dancing	Ice skating
Tennis	Canoeing (4 mph)
Jogging (4 mph)	Cycling (10 mph)
Gardening	

HEAVY WORK (energy use 7.5-9.9 calories/minute)

Jogging (5 mph)	Rugby football
Soccer	Gymnastics
Hockey	Country dancing
Horse riding	Swimming (breast/backstroke)
Basketball	

VERY HEAVY WORK (energy use greater than 10 calories/minute)

Swimming (crawl/butterfly)	Hill climbing
Cross country running	Rowing
Squash	Skiing
Cycling (14 mph)	

Remember that these values are an approximate guide only and will vary with your skill and the level of the competition.

Fig. 9 Energy expenditure of various activities.

'hypo'. I must stress that this is only an *approximate* guide and some trial and error is involved. The type of carbohydrate is also important as this will affect the speed at which glucose is absorbed from the intestine and enters the bloodstream.

The type of carbohydrate eaten also affects performance and the most sensible approach to strenuous activities is to take extra carbohydrate in a form that enables rapid transfer of glucose to the bloodstream for use as energy.

Although we know roughly how many calories a particular form of exercise uses up, it does vary from person to person. I would suggest at least 20g or 40g carbohydrate be eaten before a strenuous game. The effectiveness of this measure can be checked by performing a blood glucose test, say at half-time of a football match. If necessary extra carbohydrate can be eaten then.

In my experience, summer camps organised by the Youth Department of the British Diabetic Association or some of the parent/child weekends provide a unique setting where qualified help is always at hand and the newly diagnosed diabetic child or teenager can learn how to cope practically with a problem such as how much extra carbohydrate to take to prevent a 'hypo' during a football match or swimming session. You can read more about these camps in Chapter 6. Another good source of help is from other people with diabetes who you can meet at the clinic or at the local B.D.A. branch meetings.

A common problem which I have encountered in looking after people in my own clinic and also those at summer camps is the delayed 'hypo'. This occurs sometimes several hours after exercise. I remember in particular a young housewife who wanted to get back into physical trim after having had her first baby. She decided to go with her non-diabetic friend to an aerobics dancing class. The class was held between three and four o'clock in the afternoon. As she knew about the need for extra carbohydrate to cover her increased activity she ate a bag of potato crisps (32g carbohydrate; 245 calories) on the way to the hall where the classes were held. Her friend drove her home afterwards and she prepared the evening meal in the usual way. She ate this meal at a quarter to seven in the evening, having previously had her evening injection, a mixture of soluble and isophane insulin, at a quarter past six.

At around ten o'clock that night her husband noticed that she was somewhat quieter than usual and was slightly sweaty. He is an experienced 'diabetic husband' and suggested that she might be having a 'hypo' which she denied. He, of course, ignored this and persuaded her to take a glass of Coca Cola which resulted in rapid relief of her symptoms.

This case history illustrates rather well the problem of delayed 'hypo'. I discussed the 'hypo' with her at her routine clinic appointment, which fortunately came before the next weekly aerobics session. She could not think of an explanation for the 'hypo' she had experienced, not having related it to the aerobics class.

Aerobic dance classes involve quite strenuous exercise, using approximately 400 calories in half an hour, and it is after this sort of strenuous exercise that delayed 'hypos' tend to occur. For future aerobics class days my patient took an extra 10g carbohydrate mid-evening snack and was not troubled again with a 'hypo'. It is not only important to take extra carbohydrate prior to strenuous exercise but also afterwards, as the body replaces its stores of glycogen.

For more prolonged but less strenuous activities, such as gardening, playing cricket, hill walking and long shopping trips, a different approach to carbohydrate intake is needed. Because the exercise is less arduous the immediate availability of glucose from rapidly absorbed carbohydrate is not required. Additional carbohydrate is needed but it can be taken in the more usual form, that is as digestive biscuits, a wholemeal sandwich or fruit. The absorption of glucose into the blood from these types of snacks is slower but more prolonged and therefore is suitable to cover this sort of activity. Again, the effects need to be monitored and blood glucose testing should be performed, as detailed on pages 33–5.

Occasionally, despite taking adequate precautions during and after sport, 'hypos' occur even in experienced people, including medical doctors who are diabetic. In his book, *A Diabetic Doctor Looks at Diabetes: His and Yours*, Dr Peter Lodewick, who is a diabetic consultant in New Jersey, America, describes an incident which happened while he was playing tennis. Dr Lodewick is a keen advocate of sport and exercise for his diabetic patients. He also practises what he preaches and has calculated that he jogs regularly over 650 miles per year, and plays competitive tennis.

When Dr Lodewick was playing tennis on one occasion he was well up on his opponent, having won the first set 6–0 and leading 3–0 in the second. Suddenly he was overcome with weakness and his legs began to wobble. His tennis deteriorated dramatically and his opponent quickly went 4–3 up in the next set. Fortunately, Dr Lodewick's wife was watching the match and noticed the sudden change in fortune. She hinted to her husband that his blood glucose might be on the low side and provided him with a glucose-rich drink of Coke which quickly restored his former tennis prowess and he went on to win the match.

This story serves to illustrate how important it is for the diabetic person playing sport to tell team-mates, coach, school teacher or anyone else who is around during the particular activity about his or her diabetes. I know that the tendency is for most people to try to conceal illness. Because of their natural reticence, they do not want to be considered 'out of the ordinary' in any way. For the person with diabetes this is just not acceptable. A quiet word to the appropriate people at work or at play will ensure that, in the unfortunate event of a bad 'hypo', someone will be there to help. Obviously, it is important to tell these people what to do well in advance. Advise them of your particular 'hypo' symptoms and that occasionally you might be 'stroppy' during a 'hypo'; show them where you carry your Dextrosol tablets and tell them what to do if you become unconscious during a 'hypo'.

INSULIN DOSAGE

The important point with regard to insulin and exercise in the person with diabetes is worth repeating here. Once you have given an insulin injection under the skin the insulin will continue to be absorbed into the bloodstream. Whether your blood glucose level is high or low and whether you are exercising or resting has little effect on this. In the non-diabetic, insulin levels are very low during exercise whereas in the person with diabetes insulin levels may be inappropriately high. I have described how to overcome the problem by taking extra carbohydrate, but it is also possible to alter the insulin dosage.

Changing the insulin dosage can be a very effective way of avoiding hypoglycaemia during exercise and sport, but needs to be planned well in advance. If you know that on a particular day you will be involved in a prolonged sporting activity then it is possible to make some appropriate adjustment to the insulin dose. Of course, if you decide on the spur of the moment that you would like to go swimming or you are asked to join a friend in a game of tennis or squash this is not possible, especially if you are taking just two injections of insulin a day. With the insulin regimes that require smaller but more frequent injections it may still be possible to make some adjustment to the insulin. If you are taking an insulin injection before lunch, for example, you could reduce it if you have decided to play sport in the afternoon.

Often the people that I look after who go on summer camps or other sporting holidays, for instance skiing in the winter or windsurfing in the summer, reduce their insulin dosage for the period of the holiday. They know that their energy expenditure will be consistently higher during an active holiday.

The amount by which you lower the insulin will vary for particular activities and between different people. It is impossible to give detailed guidelines and you will learn by experience what is right for you. It will be helpful to hear about other people's experiences and I suggest you read Chapter 9. In addition, there are some general points that will help in your planning.

An important point is the timing of your sport and exercise in relation to your insulin injection. Think when the particular insulins you use will be having their greatest effect. One of the commonest insulin regimes is a mixture of a short- and intermediate-acting insulin given before breakfast and before the evening meal. On this regime the glucose level in the blood will be affected mainly by the short-acting insulin during the morning, and the intermediate-acting insulin in the afternoon. If you are planning sport in the morning it is reasonable to lower the quick-acting insulin. If the sport is to take place in the afternoon it is reasonable to lower the intermediate-acting insulin. The reduction in insulin dosage required will vary but for a not too competitive football match, for instance 20 per cent less insulin may be necessary.

The problem of the inappropriately high blood insulin levels for the sporting diabetic may be helped by timing of sport or exercise. Insulin levels are going to be lowest in the blood just before the next insulin injection is due. Certainly, one of my patients has found that the timing of her game of squash is crucial. The best time is late afternoon before her second injection. Of course, it is important to take extra carbohydrate at this time as well, but the relatively low insulin levels have enabled her to take part in a very energetic sport.

With regard to timing of exercise and sport some researchers have found that the blood glucose level after breakfast, which is generally the most difficult to control, is helped by exercise immediately after the meal. However, this is only feasible for those who can spare the time.

BLOOD GLUCOSE LEVELS

The thoughts that occupy the minds of most insulin-taking people when they are considering participating in sporting activities are generally related to the avoidance of hypoglycaemia. The benefits of regular exercise and sport to overall diabetic control are another important consideration. However, it is important to point out here that exercise and sport are not alternatives to good diabetic control with diet and insulin. Exercise may help control, but you must not think that as you perform sport and exercise there is no need to take the usual care with diet, insulin injections and monitoring diabetic control with blood glucose tests. The reason I stress this point, is that if your diabetes is poorly controlled, exercise can actually be dangerous because it can sometimes put the blood glucose up. In addition, and perhaps of more importance, exercise can actually cause ketosis which, as previously mentioned, is very serious and usually requires admission to hospital.

Do not be alarmed; the problem can be avoided if you know the situations in which sport can have such an effect, and you can enjoy your sporting activities without worry. The problem has been apparent for many years and is illustrated in some early studies with diabetic people in America. In 1936, Dr Marble and Dr Smith who were working at the clinic in Boston, directed by the famous American diabetologist, Dr Elliot P. Joslin, performed experiments in which they looked at the effects of exercise on blood glucose levels in people with diabetes under differing conditions. They chose young diabetic patients who were in good physical condition for their tests, which were performed first thing in the morning before breakfast. Three sorts of exercise were involved: running at a set rate, using a rowing machine and stair climbing. Blood glucose measurements were carried out regularly during the experiments.

Some of the volunteers undertook exercise without having their morning dose of insulin with breakfast. The blood glucose level in one of the volunteers, which was moderately high before exercise at about 16 mmol/l, rose to over 23 mmol/l. On another day the same person sat quietly rather than exercising during the morning, again not having had his insulin. Interestingly, his blood glucose did not rise to the same extent as after exercise. In conditions of poor control and inadequate insulin, it is apparent that exercise can actually raise the blood glucose level. These findings were also seen in another four volunteers who took part in the study. A 13 year old boy started the experiment with a blood glucose level of about 23 mmol/l which is quite high, and this went up further to about 27 mmol/l after exercise.

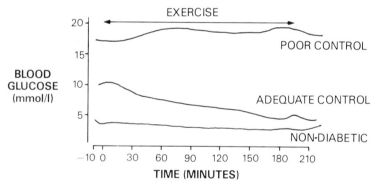

Fig. 10a The effects of exercise on blood glucose levels in diabetic people with poor control compared with those with adequate control. The blood glucose level rises slightly during exercise in the poorly controlled diabetics.
(Redrawn from Berger et al, *Diabetologia*, 13 355 (1977))

Similar studies to these pioneering efforts have been performed in more recent years and have confirmed the early findings. Included in these studies is new information which is just as important as the effects of exercise on blood glucose in the presence of poorly controlled diabetics. The information is in relation to the effect of exercise on the levels of ketones in the blood. I have plotted these results along with the glucose levels in Figs. 10a and 10b. A period of exercise in a group of people with

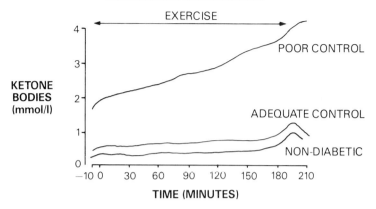

EXERCISE IN THE DIABETIC

Fig. 10b The effect of prolonged exercise on blood ketone levels in diabetics with poor control compared with those with adequate control. There is a large rise in ketones in the poorly controlled group. (Redrawn from Berger et al, *Diabetologia, 13* 355 (1977))

poor control not only produced a rise in blood glucose but also in ketones. Ketones accumulate in the blood when there is a lack of insulin, which leads to a failure of glucose uptake by body tissues and a switch to the breakdown of fat for fuel supply. Ketones are the end products of fat metabolism. These substances make the blood very acid and if severe lead to diabetic coma. When there is poor control, due to insufficient insulin, exercise can make the situation worse as the graph shows. It is likely that other hormone changes which take place on exercise, such as rises in adrenaline, cortisol, glucagon and growth hormone, as well as the insulin deficiency, contribute to the ketosis and rise in glucose.

These problems which I have just described do not affect the person who is well controlled and who wants to take part in vigorous exercise and sport. So, if you want to participate safely make sure your diabetic control is good. Exercise is no substitute for proper regard to insulin and diet in your diabetic control.

4
IMPORTANT POINTS TO NOTE

'HYPOS' IN THE OPEN AIR

For those of you who enjoy outdoor sport and activities it is important to be aware of a particular danger of 'hypos' if they occur in cold weather. This may happen, for instance, on winter sports holidays, during team sports, such as soccer or rugby, or when orienteering and fell walking. The particular danger of a 'hypo' in these situations is that the low blood glucose may interfere with the maintenance of the normal body temperature.

You will have experienced shivering, perhaps when standing waiting for a bus on an especially cold winter's day. Shivering is one of the ways the body tries to maintain normal body temperature in cold surroundings. If the body temperature falls significantly below the normal level of 37°C the condition of hypothermia may develop. The importance to the sporting and outdoor active person with diabetes is that a 'hypo' may interfere with this normal reflex of shivering in response to cold.

A series of experiments by a British researcher illustrates this point. He put volunteers who were not diabetic into a sufficiently cold environment to produce constant shivering. Insulin was then given into a vein through a drip. It was observed that when the blood glucose fell to 'hypo' levels of around 2.5–2.7 mmol/l shivering stopped. Another interesting point to emerge was that when the shivering stopped, as a result of the 'hypo', the volunteers lost their awareness of cold. When glucose was given to the volunteers through the drip to raise the blood glucose again shivering restarted.

Why a 'hypo' has this effect on shivering is not fully understood but the fact that it does should be known to all people with diabetes, their friends, families and teachers. In addition to the effect on shivering, 'hypos' cause heat loss from the body through sweating and dilating of the blood vessels in the skin.

The importance of this to the diabetic is described in a case history by Dr Hillson, a doctor experienced in looking after young adult diabetics at outward bound centres. In a report in *Diabetes Care*, an American journal devoted to diabetes research, Dr Hillson described what happened to a 17 year old diabetic girl following a mountain walk. The girl was treated with twice daily injections of a mixture of quick- and intermediate-acting insulins and, on the morning of the walk, she had reduced her morning dose of insulin by eight units and eaten twice her usual breakfast carbohydrate portions. There was heavy rain and strong wind but the group were well clothed with waterproof and wind-proof clothing and of course supervised by trained personnel. When the group returned to camp the girl went to her tent to eat some sandwiches. Some few minutes later she was found to be unconscious and was very cold. A Dextrosol glucose tablet was held against her open mouth so that some of the glucose could be absorbed into her bloodstream and within 2 minutes she started shivering and then regained consciousness, complaining bitterly of the cold. She was warmed up, given a hot meal, put in a sleeping bag and quickly recovered.

The danger of exposure should be borne in mind by everyone engaged in outdoor sport and activities in cold weather. Adequate warm waterproof and wind-proof clothing is essential, together with good waterproof footwear. Remember that the temperature falls with increasing altitude and, although the weather may be warm and sunny in the valley, it may be quite chilly up on the fells and hills. A space blanket is always a useful thing to carry in your rucksack as this will help to retain body heat in an emergency. The diabetic person is particularly at risk because of the possible effects of a 'hypo' on body temperature regulation. Therefore, if you are taking part in outdoor activities in cold weather, ensure that you have adequate clothing. If hypoglycaemia does occur then prompt action is required to raise the blood glucose. In addition, heat loss must be prevented to ensure that the body temperature does not drop to dangerous levels.

The description of these problems may be somewhat frightening but forewarned is forearmed! The type of activity where this problem may arise, such as fell walking, should not be undertaken without proper planning and supervision, and never by a diabetic person alone. However, if good preparation is made and the necessary precautions taken then problems will be rare and quickly remedied.

FOOT CARE

Anyone who has taken part in active sport or exercise may have painful memories of foot problems. The causes may have been numerous but in the most part could probably have been avoided. Problems arise from inappropriate and ill-fitting footwear. It is important that the person with diabetes should take particular care to ensure adequate foot care during exercise. After many years of diabetes, complications may develop and the feet may be affected by several of these. First of all, some nerve damage can occur in longstanding diabetes and an early feature of this nerve damage, and often the only one, is lack of normal sensation in the feet. The feet feel numb and the complaint is often described as feeling like walking on cotton wool.

Sometimes attention is drawn to the possibility of nerve damage by an ulcer or blister appearing on the foot caused by pressure from ill-fitting shoes. Because normal sensation is impaired there may be no pain. The feet may also be affected by poor blood circulation. Both the larger blood vessels (arteries) and small blood vessels (capillaries) can be affected in longstanding diabetes. If the feet are affected by both nerve damage and poor circulation, then particular care is required. If blood glucose levels are not well controlled healing of blisters or sores on the feet is impaired and infection likely.

These complications are much less likely to occur in diabetic people who have good glucose control, and attention to the feet from the moment the condition is diagnosed may help prevent problems arising later on. For this reason I have listed some do's and don'ts aimed at enabling you to perform proper foot care (see Figs. 11a and 11b).

Time and thought must be given to the choice of suitable footwear. The type will, of course, depend on the sport involved. It is important to remember that 'sports' shoes' are not necessarily interchangeable and those suitable for tennis may

IMPORTANT POINTS TO NOTE

DOs

1. Take care of your feet, they are very important; inspect them every day and always wear clean well-fitting cotton or wool socks and well-fitting leather shoes, preferably lace-up style. Feel inside the shoes to make sure that there are no rough edges.

2. Keep your feet clean; wash them every day in lukewarm water with a mild soap. Dry your feet carefully with a soft towel and remember to dry between the toes, then dust with talcum powder.

3. Cut your toe-nails carefully after washing which makes the nails softer. Cut straight across the nail but not too close to the skin as shown in the picture.

4. If dry skin is a problem, use a moisturizing cream or lotion, such as lanolin, after washing. Avoid applying lotion between the toes.

5. If you develop problems with your feet, such as callouses, ingrowing toenails and corns, see the clinic chiropodist as soon as possible. The chiropodist can also give useful advice on the prevention of damage to the feet.

DON'Ts

1. Never walk barefoot or wear socks that pinch as this can lead to ulcers.

2. Never use hot water bottles on the feet.

3. Never soak your feet for a long time in hot water as this can damage the skin.

4. Never treat your own corns, ingrowing toe-nails, etc. This is for the expert chiropodist to do. Never ever apply strong antiseptics or adhesive dressing to the feet.

Fig. 11a Do's and don'ts of foot care.

not be suitable for running. Good sports shops stock footwear specifically designed for different sporting activities and should be able to give advice.

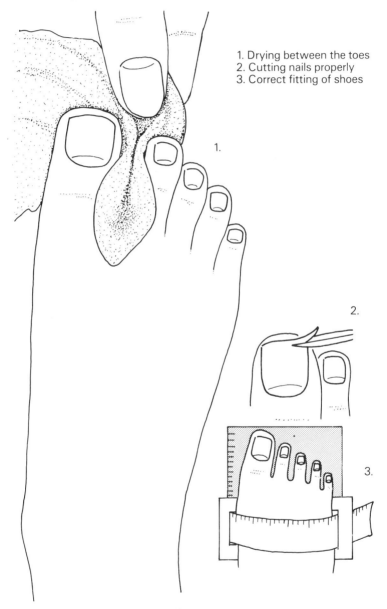

1. Drying between the toes
2. Cutting nails properly
3. Correct fitting of shoes

Fig. 11b

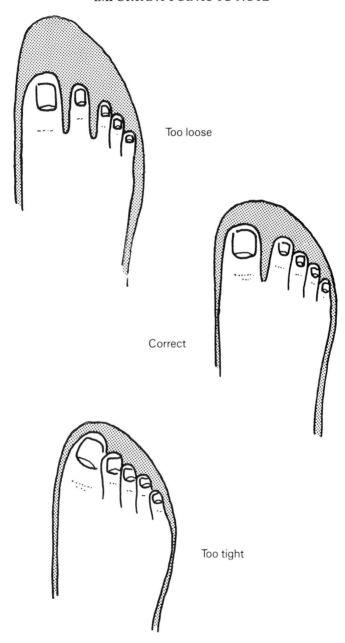

Too loose

Correct

Too tight

Fig. 12 Ensure that shoes fit correctly and comfortably.

In general, the shoe or boot should be well fitting, not too tight or too loose (see Fig. 12). There should be enough room for the toes, so that they are not cramped together and that they lie in their normal positions. Feel inside the shoes to make sure that there are no parts that are likely to rub and cause blisters. Soft leather is better for sports boots than plastic, as the leather allows the feet to 'breathe', i.e., the feet remain cooler and perspire less.

Socks are as important and should be made of cotton or wool. Again, the socks should not cramp the toes. They should be changed each day, and socks with seams or darns or elastic tops are best avoided.

Another potential hazard to the feet for the person who plays sport is athlete's foot, which can cause considerable discomfort. This is in fact the commonest fungal infection of the skin and can be caused by a variety of organisms. It tends to occur amongst people who share communal washing facilities and is therefore common in schools and sports clubs. The first thing to look for is scaling and cracking of the skin webs between the toes, and it usually affects one foot more than the other. Athlete's foot is worse in warm weather and may spread to involve all the toes with blister formation. The blisters and areas between the toes can get infected with bacteria and if not treated severe infection of the skin can result.

The fungi like warm, moist conditions, so make sure that feet are dried with a clean towel very thoroughly, especially between the toes. Talcum powder is helpful in keeping the area between the toes dry. I generally recommend a dusting powder containing a substance active against fungi, such as Mycil powder. If you are unfortunate and do get a bad fungal infection of the feet then your doctor will be able to treat this with drugs and ointments, and any secondary infection with antibiotics. Occasionally, infection spreads from the feet to the groins, so pay particular attention to these areas when showering and changing after sport, making sure that they are thoroughly dry and use dusting powder.

ALCOHOL

The soccer and rugby teams I played for at college were absolutely pitiful. They were the third or fourth teams put out by the college each week and the captains were grateful for anyone who could actually stand up! Most of the players were not particularly interested in the games and on some Saturday afternoons in mid-winter would have much preferred to be in front of the television. The big attraction for most of the players was the entertainment after the match. The fixtures included a lot of games against what are called 'social sides', that is perhaps the third team put out by an old boys' association or a work's team. The members of these teams were also just as interested in what happened after the match as in the match itself.

After the game both teams would retire, nursing their bruises and trying to recover their breath, to a suitable local hostelry where all the good of their rather pitiful attempts at exercise would be undone by 2 or 3 hours of steady beer drinking. Each team member, referee and linesman put money in a kitty and beer was consumed by the jugful until the kitty ran out. The point of this rather rambling tale is to highlight the potential dangers of alcohol to the person with diabetes. I do not advise my patients against taking alcoholic drinks and alcohol is really no less suitable for insulin taking people than for anybody else. However, a sensible approach is required, particularly after rigorous exercise of any kind. The problem is that excessive amounts of alcohol can actually affect the ability of the body to produce its own supply of glucose. You will remember that the body's supply of glucose comes not only from the diet but also from the liver where it is made by a process called gluconeogenesis. As already emphasised, this metabolic process is very important for the supply of glucose to the bloodstream for use as a fuel by important body tissues such as the brain. Alcohol can interfere with the activity of this process and increase the risk of a 'hypo'. A 'hypo' after alcohol is also potentially more serious because the body's natural defences are impaired. The blocking of gluconeogenesis by alcohol is even more significant if the amount of glucose stored in the liver as glycogen is low, such as after a prolonged period of sport. To emphasize my point, it is worth telling you that non-diabetics who have not eaten well for a few days can develop a 'hypo' after an alcohol 'binge'.

High levels of alcohol in the blood affect the function of the brain and can cause slurring of the speech, loss of balance and confusion. If you have these symptoms after drinking too much alcohol, it may be difficult for your friends to know whether you are 'hypo' or 'tipsy'. Some of my patients have been arrested for being drunk and disorderly, when really they had only consumed a small amount of alcohol. They had had a 'hypo', producing symptoms similar to those of being drunk. A policeman seeing this behaviour and smelling the alcohol had no doubt about the problem and the patients were promptly arrested. Fortunately, the mistake was spotted very soon because they were carrying identity bracelets clearly marked and stating 'I am a diabetic'.

The answer is to avoid these problems by moderation. There is no reason why you should not enjoy a pint (and I stress *a* pint) at the club, or in the pub after sport but do not 'binge'. Remember that the so-called special diabetic lager or beer which is counted as 'free' on the diet sheet because it contains hardly any carbohydrate is stronger than ordinary beer because the carbohydrate has been converted into alcohol.

5

SPORTS TO AVOID

Most doctors, including myself, who look after people with diabetes help and encourage their patients to lead a full and active life. Modern diabetic treatment is directed to this end, as well as to achieving the best possible control of blood glucose. However, there are certain sports and pastimes which I feel are best avoided by the person on insulin. All of us at some time dream of sailing round the world, climbing in the Himalayas or driving a formula one racing car round Brands Hatch etc., but have to console ourselves and apply our enthusiasm and energy to things that are within our reach.

The guiding principle in deciding which sports and pastimes are best avoided by the person on insulin is whether there is any danger to the individual concerned, or to others involved in that sport. The danger arises, of course, from the rapid development of a 'hypo'. If unexpected hypoglycaemia occurs then the safety of others as well as the person on insulin may be at risk. All people with diabetes deciding on any sporting activity must be aware of the symptoms of a 'hypo', as even the best controlled person may experience this. Hence the additional safety measures, described on page 31, are necessary.

In my opinion, pastimes involving the control of a powerful vehicle, such as motor racing, motorbike racing, motor cross, power boat driving etc., are not advisable. In the event of a 'hypo', and if the vehicle went out of control, the obvious danger would be to passengers or spectators. Piloting any sort of aircraft is out for the person on insulin, and hang-gliding similarly. Mountaineering and rock climbing are generally not suitable. However, at some of the B.D.A. summer camps rock climbing and abseiling have been included in the activities available. These activities were, of course, very carefully supervised by skilled youth leaders, together with nurses and a doctor, who were in continual attendance.

A colleague of mine was supervising a session of abseiling at an adventure centre on the south coast. One of the boys had a rapid severe 'hypo' while in the middle of his abseil and began to have convulsions, which sometimes accompany a bad 'hypo'. However, there was absolutely no danger to the boy as there was an additional safety rope attached to him and controlled by an experienced youth leader who quickly lowered him the 15 feet or so to the bottom of the rock face where my colleague administered an intravenous glucose injection. This quickly restored him and he was happy to continue. I do not include fell walking as being unsuitable but special precautions are necessary (see page 53).

In 1982, I remember seeing an article in *Balance*, the newspaper of the British Diabetic Association. (This newspaper is received free of charge by members of the British Diabetic Association and the majority of my patients have at some time derived great benefit from its articles.) The story revolved around a 26 year old man with diabetes (the condition had developed when he was 13 years old), who had joined an expedition travelling to the Far East and Australia to explore and photograph coral reefs.

The article was very interesting and described the expedition in great detail. However, it did point out the hazards of sub-aqua diving (using compressed air cylinders) for people on insulin. In fact, the present ruling of the British Sub-Aqua Club is that those with insulin dependent diabetes, however well controlled or fit, should not be allowed to dive. The reason for this is best explained by a quotation from a letter published in the *British Medical Journal* on 3 October 1981, from the medical adviser to the Sub-Aqua Association. He was concerned about the numbers of diabetic people diving for pleasure, having been assured by their medical advisers that there was nothing to worry about. He pointed out that people with diabetes were excluded from being professional divers and the policy of the Sub-Aqua Association was that they should not dive. The main problem is that of hypoglycaemia, and the increased risks associated with a 'hypo' when it occurs underwater. The combination of a 'hypo' with decompression sickness is particularly hazardous. Snorkel diving is not as dangerous as sub-aqua or scuba diving and is quite possible for people with diabetes, so long as adequate precautions are taken.

The August, 1983, edition of *Balance* had a picture on the front page showing a 52 year old insulin taking housewife about to start a sailing trip around the world. However, she was not going to do this alone but with her husband and two grown up children. She was well prepared for the trip and their sailing ketch was equipped with a special medical fridge to house a year's supply of insulin plus some other medical provisions including glucagon. 'Hypos' occasionally happened when she was tired but both her husband and daughter knew how to inject her with glucagon.

I prefer to make this chapter as short as possible, as it is somewhat negative to discuss those activities which are not recommended for diabetics. To sum up, fell walking, sailing, swimming in the sea, water sports, orienteering, canoeing and hiking amongst other sports should not be carried out alone. On the other hand, if the person on insulin is with a group and that group know about the condition and how to cope in the unlucky event of a 'hypo', then these activities can be safely undertaken.

6

BRITISH DIABETIC ASSOCIATION SUMMER CAMPS

In many parts of this book I mention the British Diabetic Association (B.D.A.) and the summer camps which it organises. The importance which I attach to the Association and its youth work is emphasised by the fact that I have devoted a chapter solely to its activities.

I want to concentrate particularly on the youth work of the Association but would also like to mention the general importance of the B.D.A. The benefits which the B.D.A. has provided for the person with diabetes over the years are incalculable. The Association gives advice on all aspects of diabetic life through its various publications and its newspaper, *Balance* is excellent and open to all for a nominal membership fee.

The local B.D.A. branches provide a forum for discussion of the problems concerned with diabetic life, and introductions for the newly diagnosed in a particular area. This enables the person new to diabetes and their family to draw on a wealth of invaluable experience. Another important feature of the Association's activities is its support for research into diabetes. As a young doctor I was awarded a scholarship from the Association and I am very grateful for the opportunity this gave me to develop an interest and perform research into diabetes.

Doctors and scientists interested in diabetes are not only general members of the Association but also members of the Medical and Scientific Section. This section organises two meetings each year where physicians and scientists meet to discuss their research work into the disease. About five hundred people attend these meetings, which contribute to the general standard of diabetic care by training young doctors to become specialists in diabetes and also by keeping the established diabetic consultants up-to-date with new developments.

It is the youth work of the Association upon which I wish to concentrate, with special emphasis on the summer camps. I am very grateful to the Youth Department of the B.D.A., for providing me with up-to-date information about camp activities to supplement my own experience over the last ten years. The ability to cope with sport and outdoor activities is inseparable from general diabetic education. There are several useful publications to help with general education (see 'Suggested Further Reading') but there is no substitute for practical experience and the summer camps are a wonderful way of learning to cope with everyday situations under expert guidance and tuition. I should point out also that the camps also provide an excellent holiday!

The camps, in their present form, have been running since 1952. In that period, over 9000 children and young adults with diabetes have benefited from attending one or more camps. Sometimes those who originally attended camps as children return in later years as members of the staff. The staffing of the camps is very important and includes doctors, nurses and dieticians, as well as leaders. For a junior camp consisting of about forty children there would usually be two doctors, two or three nurses, two or three dieticians and about eight leaders, together with the camp warden. You will note that the ratio of staff to children is high, thereby allowing close supervision when necessary.

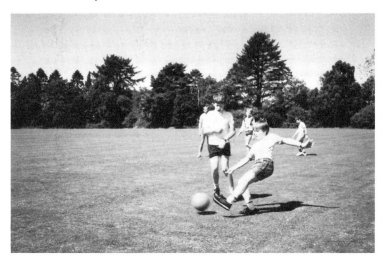

There are many things to be learned by the newly diagnosed. It can be an overwhelming experience for the child and the parents to begin with, and it is easy to see why it is so daunting. There are not only the problems of insulin injection technique, measuring the correct dose of insulin, understanding of the diabetic diet, blood and urine testing and the problems of hypoglycaemia, but also other less obvious areas, such as meals out, day trips away from home, parties, sports, games and P.E. lessons at school.

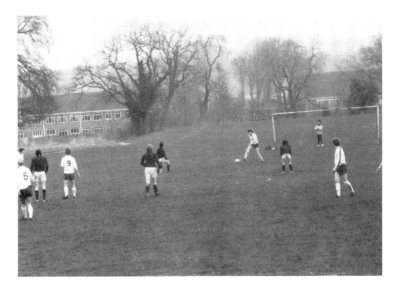

Along with these practical skills and knowledge, the person with diabetes has to come to terms with the condition and become confident and self-reliant. Lack of self-confidence, repeated hospital admission (which can be avoided), unnecessary restrictions at home or school (for instance with regard to sport) damage self-esteem and can cause unhappiness.

The camps play a very important role in helping young people to learn about and conquer everyday problems of the diabetic life. Many children at these camps have told me how pleased they were to meet others with diabetes and to learn from them as well as the staff. However, from what I have said do not imagine that these camps resemble school! First and foremost the participants get a terrific holiday and formal teaching is at most a couple of hours during the week. Problems such as how to cope with a game of football or disco dancing, in terms of additional carbohydrate intake and insulin dosage, can be dealt with on an individual basis because of the large number of qualified staff available.

The camps demonstrate that it is possible to take part in the majority of activities. They point out that although diabetes cannot be forgotten the burden is not intolerable. It must be difficult for some parents to think of allowing their son or daughter to leave home for a couple of weeks, but the standard of care at the camps with experienced doctors and nurses always directly available must be reassuring. The change in a young person after only one camp can be quite dramatic. Someone who was perhaps shy and retiring and reluctant to take part in games and group activities for fear of hypoglycaemia can only gain from the experience of the camp, and will return home more confident and self-reliant.

JUNIOR CAMPS

The camps are organised in such a way that the children attending a particular camp are about the same age. For the younger age groups 5–6, 7–8, 8–9, 9–11, 9–12 and 12–15 years there are about 15 camps held in the school holidays. They are situated at sites all over Britain, ranging from Cobham in Kent to Dunkeld in Perthshire, and from Llandrindod Wells in Powys to Blythburgh in Suffolk. Although called camps, in fact most are not held under canvas but in schools etc., however the Spring-hill camps are real camping holidays.

Obviously, more staff are needed to look after the younger children some of whom have had diabetes for only a very short time. Close supervision is given to insulin injections, diet and blood or urine testing. Children previously unable to give their own injections go away quite confident in injection techniques at the end of the camp. At camps, amongst other points, rotation of the injection site is encouraged and children may be introduced to the new 'microfine' disposable syringes, if they are not already familiar with them. These make injections much more comfortable.

Blood glucose testing at home is a tremendous aid to good diabetic control and even young children are able to do this. It can be done painlessly and accurately by a relatively simple procedure, and provides much more valuable information than urine testing. It is easily taught at the camp.

Attention is paid to diet for the juniors and as wide a range of foods as possible is provided at meal times to help the children increase their understanding of carbohydrate exchanges. Account is now taken of the new B.D.A. dietary recommendations and the children are encouraged to try high fibre foods, such as wholemeal bread, wholewheat cereals and plenty of fresh fruit and vegetables. High fibre foods aid diabetic control as they produce slower increases in blood glucose. Foods with a high sugar content are generally avoided but they can be used, for instance, to supply the additional carbohydrate (for example, chocolate biscuits) prior to sport. Excess animal fat in the diet is generally discouraged. There are tuck shops at the junior camps where special diabetic sweets and chocolates can be bought together with low calorie canned drinks.

The activities on the junior camps vary but to give you some idea I will tell you a little about the camp held at the Purbeck Centre, Swanage. The camp, held in a converted school with good facilities, is for children aged between ten and twelve. The centre is quite large and other youth groups such as cub packs tend to be there at the same time. This provides the diabetic children with the opportunity to meet other children, and games such as football can be organised with teams drawn from the different groups.

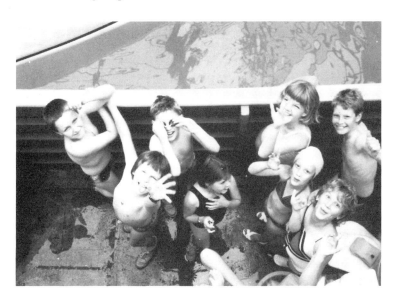

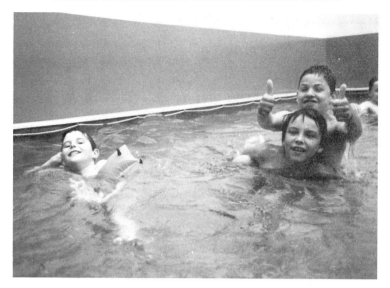

The centre has dormitory accommodation with bunk beds for the children and there is plenty of space for indoor activities such as table tennis and discos. A heated outdoor swimming pool is popular and used very often. Other outdoor activities include football and rounders, treasure hunts, sports days and swimming galas. For these events the children are divided into teams – Tigers, Panthers, and Lions. Many excursions are arranged and the children at one camp had a ride on a troop landing craft, courtesy of the Royal Marines at a local base. Other trips take in Corfe Castle, a tank museum at an army camp, an agricultural college and farm where cows are seen being milked, Brownsea Island in Poole Harbour, local beaches, and shopping expeditions. During one camp the Radio One Roadshow visited Swanage and the children went along and had a dedication played over the radio.

TEENAGE CAMPS

The Association also organises camps for teenage diabetics in the age ranges 13–18, 14–16, 14–17 and 16–25. I have personal experience of these camps and they offer a wide range of opportunities. People attending the teenage camps tend to have had diabetes for longer and generally have more experience in managing their condition. However, as with the juniors, it is

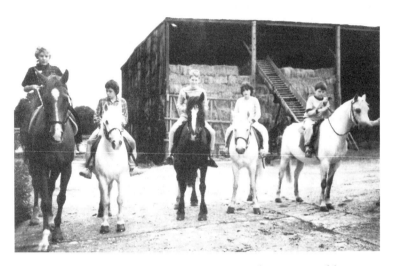

often possible to iron out injection technique problems to increase understanding of diet and to encourage home monitoring of blood glucose, etc.

It is my practice, having identified problems, to try to solve them on an individual basis and this seems to work well. The rapport which develops at the camps through sharing of accommodation, activities and meals and the informal atmosphere often enables long-standing problems of diabetic management to be remedied. However, what I feel to be the real value of the camps is the opportunity provided to take part in a wide range of activities. The activities are often personally demanding (and would be for the non-diabetic) and give a tremendous sense of achievement on completion. The teenagers leave the camps confident in the knowledge and experience of how to control their diabetes in all manner of situations.

There are several regular camps organised by the B.D.A. for teenagers – ranging from Poole in Dorset to Eskdale in Cumbria. The camp in Poole is held at the Poole and Dorset Adventure Centre (age group 13–18). I acted as the medical officer on two occasions at this particular camp and I left there much fitter than when I arrived! Activities included swimming, with opportunities to practise underwater swimming, and rescue and life-saving techniques which made full use of the beautiful Poole Harbour. When I was there an excellent swimming pool at the Royal Marines base in Hamworthy was also available.

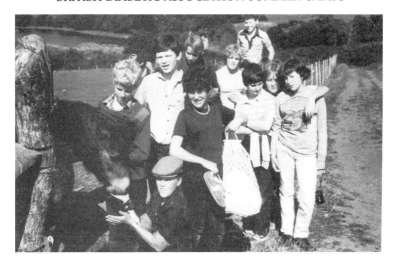

Other activities included canoeing and dinghy sailing with instruction in basic techniques. Tuition was given in map reading and camping techniques, and an important event of the week was the twelve mile hike with full kit over the Purbeck Hills, followed by an overnight camp on a site overlooking Corfe Castle. Some simple rock climbing and abseiling was available which was thoroughly enjoyed.

These activities were particularly strenuous and the necessity for extra carbohydrate and alteration in insulin dosage to cover additional exertion was soon learned. It was also important to carry suitable additional carbohydrate on long hiking and canoeing expeditions. The disposable insulin syringes made a tremendous difference on camping expeditions.

The Abernethy Outdoor Centre (age group 14–17) which was used for the first time in 1983 was very successful, and hopefully will become a regular site for a B.D.A. camp. The centre has really excellent facilities and sports equipment and is set in beautiful countryside, in a 30 acre estate close to the Cairngorm mountains. The indoor sports complex includes a squash court, a hall for basketball, volleyball, badminton or indoor soccer, and a games room for table tennis and snooker. A swimming pool is also available and outside are sports fields and an adventure course.

Outdoor activities include canoeing and sailing on the local loch (Loch Morlich); hill walking, rock climbing and abseiling in the Cairngorm mountains; and cycling and orienteering in the surrounding countryside. All the specialised equipment, including life jackets and climbing boots, are available at the centre and there is room on the camp for 30 people aged 14–17 years together with an experienced team of leaders, doctors, nurses and dieticians.

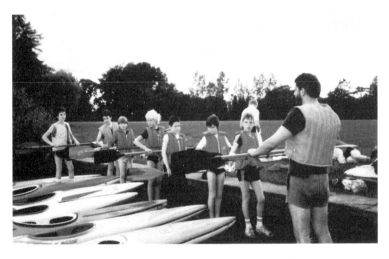

An outward bound centre provides perhaps the most taxing activities available outside the rigorous training demanded for specialised branches of the armed services. At a recent meeting of the Medical and Scientific Section of the B.D.A., Dr Hilson related the exploits of a group of thirteen insulin dependent diabetics aged 16–20 years who she looked after as Medical Officer at an outward bound centre in Eskdale, Cumbria. She illustrated her talk with magnificent photographs taken during the 12-day course. The photographs revealed the dramatic nature of some of the challenging activities available which were, of course, supervised by a highly trained team of leaders and medical staff. Everyone seemed to find the more challenging parts of the course the most enjoyable and some of the comments made by the teenagers were very illuminating. One 18 year old said 'I've liked everything so far – except the washing up. I've learned more about control and how far I can push myself'. A 17 year old said 'I don't want to be treated differently because I don't think I am different. Diabetes doesn't restrict me. I'll have a go at anything once'.

As you can imagine, each day at an outward bound centre is full of activity starting, before seven in the morning, with a swim in the tarn or a jog before breakfast and followed by rock climbing, canoeing, surfing, mountain rescue and first aid, orienteering and obstacle courses. With all this extra activity the need for additional carbohydrate was very high and it was interesting to hear that one boy had mid-meal snacks of 80g carbohydrate. In fact the average increase in daily carbohydrate was about 50g and an average decrease of insulin dosage of about 6 units per day was required.

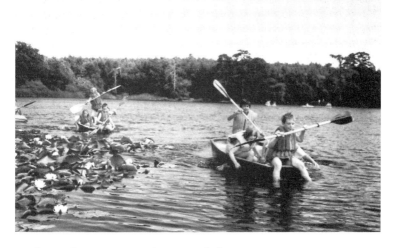

These descriptions of some of the B.D.A. camps should, if you are a young diabetic, encourage you to try one; if you are the parent of a young diabetic I hope you will be encouraged to let your son or daughter attend and feel confident that he or she is in good hands and will have an exciting and challenging time. If you are a local branch member I hope you will consider it worthwhile to sponsor your young diabetics if they cannot afford to pay the fees. (I should point out here that the fees are heavily subsidised by the B.D.A.) If you are a doctor or diabetic liaison nurse remember that a fortnight's practical experience at a camp is probably worth more to the young diabetic than any amount of advice in the clinic. If you are an older person with diabetes, who in the past attended one of these camps, think about going back as a leader and help others with your experience. The B.D.A. recently organised the first young diabetic leaders camp. This camp was designed to bring together young

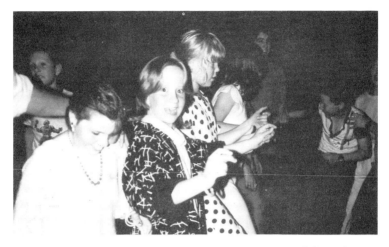

people with diabetes interested in devoting some of their time to helping other people. Ten girls and thirteen boys attended the camp which was held at the Firbush Point Field Centre on the banks of Loch Tay in Perthshire. Although there were lots of sporting opportunities for the participants including wind-surfing, sailing and white water canoeing, the main objective of the week was the discussion of the practical aspects of coping with diabetes. A group of young adults with diabetes who have encountered various pitfalls in their own diabetic lives and learned to deal with them are well qualified to render sympathetic understanding to others and help them over similar obstacles.

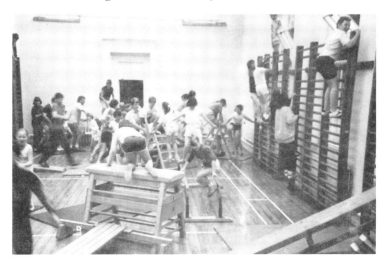

7
THE BENEFITS OF REGULAR SPORTING EXERCISE

JOSIAH MASON
COLLEGE
LIBRARY

I have explained how the body responds to exercise and how diabetes affects this response. I have done this in order to help the person with diabetes to participate in a form of activity which is tremendously enjoyable and beneficial. But what about those of you who are not keen to participate in these activities? I would like to suggest to you that there are potential benefits which might persuade you to think again. For those of you already engaged in active pursuits, are you gaining any additional benefits as well as the pleasure and fun of the sports themselves? In this chapter, I will describe some of the benefits of regular sporting exercise in relation to diabetes. Some of these benefits are still the subject of dispute amongst researchers, and further experimental studies are needed. Having said that, there is a lot of evidence to support the comments I wish to make.

DIABETIC CONTROL

In a scientific paper appearing in the *British Medical Journal*, as long ago as 10 April 1926, R. D. Lawrence stated: 'The effect of exercise in reducing blood glucose and glycosuria in diabetes mellitus has been known for many years'. He referred to the research work of Dr F. M. Allen who wrote an article in 1919 with the title *Total Dietary Regulation in the Treatment of Diabetes*. This was written before the discovery of insulin when the only treatment for diabetes was severe restriction of dietary carbohydrate. I came across a diet prescribed for a diabetic patient of

75

mine who first developed diabetes in 1916. She had the 'egg and veg' diet which consisted of green vegetables and eggs on one day, alternating with a complete fast on the next! Occasionally, depending on the blood glucose test she was allowed a very small amount of carbohydrate, such as 5oz of bread. If you as a person with diabetes in the 1980s complain about your diet, think of the restrictions in pre-insulin days! Fortunately for my patient her pancreas was obviously still producing a small amount of insulin and she survived, despite general ill health, until 1923 when she received insulin for the first time. In the pre-insulin days this diet had to be endured as it was the only treatment available. However, Dr Allen showed that exercise lowered blood glucose in all but the very severe cases. This effect was not temporary and, if the exercise was continued every day, the patient was able to take more carbohydrate in the diet without affecting the blood glucose. In fact some of these patients were only able to stay generally well and free of glycosuria if they exercised regularly.

After insulin became available for diabetic treatment in the early 1920s Dr Lawrence working with Dr G. A. Harrison, showed that exercise increased the effects of insulin on the blood glucose. They noted that symptoms of hypoglycaemia were likely to occur on days when exercise was taken if the diet and insulin were unchanged. In the paper that I have already mentioned Robin Lawrence extended his observations on the effect of exercise in insulin dependent diabetes. He illustrated this with descriptions of two patients, both young men with widely differing life styles.

The first person led a sedentary city life and was treated with twice daily insulin injections and a diet which included 45g carbohydrate per day. Dr Lawrence describes the effects of a three week holiday on this man's diabetic control. During his holiday he took frequent exercise, which was sometimes fairly strenuous in the morning, afternoon and evening. During this period he could increase his carbohydrate intake from 45 to 100g each day and his urine remained free of glucose. Ordinarily, if he added 5 or 10g carbohydrate to his diet he showed glycosuria. Lawrence commented that his patient became noticeably fatter in the face and the bulk and firmness of his muscles were greatly increased. This provides evidence that exercise enabled the same amount of insulin to metabolise a greater quantity of carbohydrate than was contained in the usual diet.

The second person worked as a gardener and the amount of his work varied considerably from time to time. His insulin requirements remained stable between October 1924 and April 1925, and his urine was free of glucose. His blood glucose measured about four hours after breakfast was very satisfactory at 5 mmol/l. From May 1925 he began to do more work and to play cricket in the evenings. Very soon a reduction in insulin dosage had to be made because of 'hypo' reactions and, by the beginning of July, his insulin requirement had decreased by nearly 40 per cent. In the middle of July, he stopped working and playing cricket and by the end of the month his blood glucose was beginning to rise and glucose appeared in the urine. Because of this his insulin dose had to be increased again.

These two case histories from the very early days of insulin therapy demonstrate the power of exercise and sport in diabetic control. Dr Lawrence stated in his paper '. . . I believe that the insulin requirements of these two cases could be interchanged by reversing their condition of life. If Case 1 adopted a life of manual labour, I feel sure that only one moderate dose of insulin would be required to keep his metabolism normal (unless his diet had to be increased to meet the increased exercise); while if Case II became sedentary in his habits he would require two moderately large doses a day, so great is the effect of exercise in aiding insulin to metabolise sugar normally'.

In recent years research scientists have carried out studies looking at the effects of physical training on insulin response and glucose metabolism, and have discovered some interesting facts in non-diabetic volunteers. This has stimulated further studies using volunteers with diabetes. It has been found that trained athletes usually have lower levels of insulin in their blood than untrained people. Despite this their blood glucose levels are entirely normal. These findings suggested to the scientists that, perhaps, insulin was more effective in athletes, i.e., a smaller amount of insulin was doing the job of maintaining normal blood glucose. An explanation soon followed when it was discovered that body tissue removed from athletes and studied in the laboratory appeared to bind more insulin.

Before insulin can exert its effects on cells it has to stick to them, a process called binding. This process can be studied in monocytes (white blood cells) using radioactive insulin. The results have led to a possible explanation for the increased sensitivity of the effects of insulin seen with physical training.

Monocytes from athletes bind more insulin than those of untrained people, which suggests that the cells have more areas available on the cell surface to which insulin can bind. These areas are called insulin receptors.

This research work has been taken further by studying volunteers before and after a period of physical training. In one particular study, performed in America at Yale University School of Medicine, six healthy men (average age 25 years) worked on an exercise bicycle for one hour, four times a week over a period of six weeks. The exercise on the bicycle was quite intense and the volunteers were performing at about two-thirds of their maximum possible capacity. Their heart rate went up to 160–170 beats each minute (normal resting rate is about 70 beats per minute). The researchers found that the amount of insulin binding to cells increased by over a third after the training programme, due to an increase in the number of insulin recptors in the cells. The research workers calculated that the number of receptors went up from about 15,000 per cell to 24,000 per cell.

As well as looking at the behaviour of these cells in the laboratory, the scientists performed tests on the volunteers before and after the 6 weeks exercise in which they obtained an assessment of glucose uptake by the whole body. These studies are a little complex but, in simple terms, insulin was given to the volunteers by a drip into a vein. This tended to reduce the blood glucose, as every person with diabetes is aware. To balance the insulin, glucose solution was given and the amount varied to keep the blood glucose constant. From the amount of glucose that had to be given to balance the effect of the insulin, the researchers could calculate how much glucose was being taken up by the body. They found that this went up by about a third after the training. The effect is probably due to increased uptake of glucose into the muscles. The results showed, therefore, that physical exercise over a period of six weeks could produce marked effects on the metabolism of insulin and glucose, suggesting that beneficial effects might be seen if diabetic people undertook regular exercise.

Some studies on insulin-taking volunteers have since been carried out. For instance, a group of researchers from Norway presented some of their work at an International Meeting on Diabetes and Exercise held in Greece in 1980. They studied six young insulin-ta... teenagers aged between 15 and 16 years. For the purpo... the experiment they undertook five exercise sessions lasting 45 minutes every day for 2 weeks. During this time their insulin dose needed to be reduced by well over a third and their blood glucose control improved significantly.

These experiments produced dramatic effects but I am not suggesting that it is necessary to exercise to such an extent to obtain a useful effect on diabetic control. Why exercise has this beneficial effect on blood glucose levels and insulin dosage has been studied and, as with non-diabetics, exercise appears to be associated with an increase in the sensitivity of body tissue to the effect of insulin. This was shown by a group of research doctors from Denmark. (Denmark as a country has made a very large contribution to diabetic research and, as I am sure you will know, produces through the Novo and Nordisk companies some of the most widely used insulins.) They performed studies on nine young men whose diabetes was well controlled. None of them was very athletic. Blood samples were taken on three different days: firstly, when they were resting; second, when they were exercising on a bicycle exercise machine for three hours after eating breakfast and taking their normal insulin; and thirdly, again first thing in the morning when they exercised on an empty stomach with no insulin injection. These studies revealed that the amount of insulin binding to cells increased during both periods of exercise. The cells used in this study to measure the insulin binding were red cells (erythrocytes) and white cells which are not involved in the body's response to exercise. However, insulin binding to these cells does seem to correlate with glucose tolerance and insulin sensitivity. Changes demonstrated in these cells may well occur in working muscles and contribute to the effect of exercise in reducing blood glucose.

Another scientific study on exercise and diabetic control, carried out by a group of researchers from Toronto, Canada, looked at the effect of exercise on the rise in blood glucose after breakfast. The volunteers performed moderate exercise for 45 minutes starting 30 minutes after breakfast. This period of exercise was sufficient to reduce the highest glucose level from 15 to 11 mmol/l.

The researchers suggested two reasons for this effect. Firstly, that the blood supply to the intestine was reduced by the exercise, resulting in a slower absorption of glucose and, secondly, that the glucose absorbed was used preferentially by the exercising muscles. The exercise taken after breakfast improved blood glucose levels after lunch as well. The finding is presumably related to the study from Denmark, which showed the increased receptors for insulin after exercise.

Although these experiments demonstrate the potential value of exercise on diabetic control, they bear little resemblance to normal daily activity. However, researchers have tried to look at the effects of regular exercise over longer time periods to see whether diabetic control is improved. One of these studies was performed by doctors in Michigan, America. Nine insulin-taking children took part in an exercise programme for 3 months. The exercise programme consisted of three 30-minute sessions each week involving running, games and movement to music. After twelve weeks the children who took part showed improved diabetic control, measured by a reduction in their glycosylated haemoglobin concentrations. These children were also physically fitter after the study. On the other hand, some researchers have not found that prolonged exercise programmes improve diabetic control and further research work needs to be performed on this topic.

WEIGHT REDUCTION

Obesity (overweight) has become a very important health problem in the western world. People who are obese have a greater risk of dying earlier. This increased risk is due mainly to heart disease but many other diseases are also more common in obese people. Exactly why obesity is associated with heart disease is not clear, but it is likely that it is due to factors associated with increased body weight, such as raised blood fat levels and raised blood pressure.

Obesity is an important problem, therefore, for the person with diabetes as well as for the non-diabetic. An additional problem in diabetes is that obesity makes the body's cells less sensitive to the action of insulin because there are fewer insulin receptors. These research findings support the experience gained from looking after overweight diabetic people who usually require more insulin.

Obese people without diabetes tend to have a lower level of physical activity than those who are not overweight. This is also seen in thin people who deliberately overeat to become fat, as part of an experiment. When these volunteers have become obese there is a reduction in and a lack of motivation to perform physical exercise. This relationship between obesity and lack of physical activity could be due to the voluntary reduction in activity by overweight people, which probably helps to perpetuate the obesity. It is also likely that overweight people with diabetes tend to have decreased physical activity, but can exercise and sport help to achieve a reduction in weight? It can help but only along with other measures and in particular a reduction in the number of calories in the diet. Exercise is certainly not effective on its own in producing weight loss but when combined with a low calorie diet it has several beneficial effects.

While advocating exercise in the obese diabetic person to aid weight loss I do not recommend a sudden start at any vigorous game or jogging ten miles a day! It is very unlikely, even with the best intentions and a lot of motivation, that the overweight person would be able to do this! More important, however, sudden vigorous exertion in the totally unfit and overweight can be dangerous. Any sort of exercise activity in this situation, particularly in the older person, should be carefully planned and discussed with the local doctor or diabetic clinic doctor. If care is taken, then a daily exercise or sport tailored to the individual can be very beneficial.

At first, the amount of physical activity should be low and it should be increased gradually as the person becomes fitter. Aerobic physical activity is the best form of exercise and walking is a convenient way to start. This should initially be limited to about a mile a day, taking perhaps half an hour to walk the distance. This level of activity should be maintained for at least a week when the amount of walking can be increased to two walks of the same distance each day, amounting to 14 miles a week. Maintain this for a further week. In the following weeks the distance walked can be progressively increased, about 2 miles a week would be reasonable. When the amount of walking has risen to about 20 miles each week, the speed of the walking can be increased to cover approximately 2 miles in half an hour. This amount of exercise will burn up about 150 calories. As fitness increases then other forms of exercise, such as swimming or cycling, can be taken up.

Again let me emphasise that physical exercise on its own will not reduce weight but must be combined with a reduction in the number of calories eaten. The ideal weight tables (for adults)

MEN

Height		Small frame		Medium frame		Large frame	
ft in	(cm)	lb	kg	lb	kg	lb	kg
5 1	(155)	112-120	(51-54)	118-129	(54-59)	126-141	(57-64)
5 2	(157)	115-123	(52-56)	121-133	(55-60)	129-144	(59-65)
5 3	(160)	118-126	(54-57)	124-136	(56-62)	132-148	(60-67)
5 4	(163)	121-129	(55-58)	127-139	(58-63)	135-152	(61-69)
5 5	(165)	124-133	(56-60)	130-143	(59-65)	138-156	(63-71)
5 6	(168)	128-137	(58-62)	134-147	(61-67)	142-161	(64-73)
5 7	(170)	132-141	(60-64)	138-152	(63-69)	147-166	(67-75)
5 8	(173)	136-145	(62-66)	142-156	(64-71)	151-170	(68-77)
5 9	(175)	140-150	(63-68)	146-160	(66-73)	155-174	(70-79)
5 10	(178)	144-154	(65-70)	150-165	(68-75)	159-179	(72-81)
5 11	(180)	148-158	(67-72)	154-170	(70-77)	164-184	(74-83)
6 0	(183)	152-162	(69-74)	158-175	(72-80)	168-189	(76-86)
6 1	(185)	156-167	(71-76)	162-180	(74-82)	173-194	(78-88)
6 2	(188)	160-171	(73-78)	167-185	(76-84)	178-199	(81-90)
6 3	(190)	164-175	(74-80)	172-190	(76-86)	182-204	(83-92)

WOMEN

Height		Small frame		Medium frame		Large frame	
ft in	(cm)	lb	kg	lb	kg	lb	kg
4 8	(142)	92-98	(42-44)	96-107	(44-49)	104-119	(47-54)
4 9	(145)	94-101	(43-46)	98-110	(45-50)	106-122	(48-55)
4 10	(147)	96-104	(44-47)	101-113	(46-51)	109-125	(49-57)
4 11	(150)	99-107	(45-48)	104-116	(47-53)	112-128	(51-58)
5 0	(152)	102-110	(46-50)	107-119	(48-54)	115-131	(52-59)
5 1	(155)	105-113	(48-51)	110-122	(50-55)	118-134	(53-60)
5 2	(157)	108-116	(49-53)	113-126	(51-57)	121-138	(55-63)
5 3	(160)	111-119	(50-54)	116-130	(53-59)	125-142	(57-64)
5 4	(163)	114-123	(52-56)	120-135	(54-61)	129-146	(58-66)
5 5	(165)	118-127	(53-58)	124-139	(56-63)	133-150	(60-68)
5 6	(168)	122-131	(55-59)	128-143	(58-65)	137-154	(62-70)
5 7	(170)	126-135	(57-61)	132-147	(60-67)	141-158	(64-72)
5 8	(173)	130-140	(59-63)	136-151	(62-69)	145-163	(66-74)
5 9	(175)	134-144	(61-65)	140-155	(63-70)	149-168	(68-76)
5 10	(178)	138-148	(63-67)	144-159	(65-72)	153-173	(69-78)

Fig. 13 Weight tables for men and women aged 25 years and over. (From the life tables of the Metropolitan Life Insurance Company of New York)

shown in Fig. 13 will help you see if you are overweight.

BLOOD FAT LEVELS

Quite understandably, the person with diabetes and his doctor tend to be preoccupied with the maintenance of near normal blood glucose concentrations and avoidance of 'hypos'. Marked variations in blood glucose can cause distressing symptoms and good long-term control of blood glucose levels is very important in preventing problems in later life. However, as you will have discovered earlier in the book, insulin not only affects the metabolism of carbohydrate but also that of fats and protein. In fact, abnormalities of blood fats are seen quite often in diabetes and are probably of importance in relation to diseases of blood vessels just as they are in non-diabetics. Newspapers and magazines often carry articles on blood fats, particularly cholesterol, but until relatively recently Britain has tended to lag behind countries like the United States in an awareness of their significance.

The most well-known of the blood fats is cholesterol. This substance is found in large amounts in the fatty deposits, known as atheroma plaques, which occur in the lining of blood vessels. These plaques are responsible for narrowing of the blood vessels, resulting in poor blood circulation to important parts of the body, such as the heart, brain and legs. The condition may lead to strokes, heart attacks and gangrene. In fact, in western developed countries, illnesses related to atheroma plaques are the commonest cause of death.

As these diseases are so much more common in developed countries, which have a higher standard of living, a reasonable assumption has been made over the years that the type of diet eaten in the West may be associated with increased heart disease. There is good evidence from large studies of different populations that this is indeed the case. The major differences in diet between rich and poor countries are the total amount of food consumed, and notably the amount of animal fat and refined carbohydrate. These are, of course, much higher in the average western diet and one of the effects of this is excess weight or obesity. Another feature of dietary excess in western countries is that the level of blood fats tends to be high.

Diabetes is associated with elevated blood fats because of the effects of insulin on fat metabolism. Until relatively recently, there was another factor of importance with regard to blood fats in diabetics and that was the dietary advice generally given in diabetic clinics. This tended to concentrate on carbohydrate restriction, with an increase in the amount of animal fat eaten to make up the calories. Most people with diabetes were probably taking even more animal fat in their diets than the already high amount taken by the average non-diabetic. The British Diabetic Association has issued new dietary guidelines which include an increase in the amount of carbohydrate (particularly with a high fibre content) in the diet and a reduction in animal fat. One of the reasons for these changes in dietary recommendations is to reduce blood fat levels.

In addition to diet the degree of blood glucose control is important in determining the level of blood fats in diabetics. In general with good diabetic control the level of blood fats tends to fall. However, a blood fat particle known as H.D.L. rises with good control and this in some way seems to protect against the development of atheroma plaques. It may do this by helping the body get rid of cholesterol.

Can regular exercise with good blood glucose control and a suitable diet help to reduce harmful blood fat levels? Certainly, in non-diabetics there is a large amount of evidence to suggest that those who undertake regular physical exercise have lower levels of blood fat particles, and higher levels of H.D.L. These findings have been shown in long distance skiers, joggers running more than 25 km/week, tennis players and marathon runners. Those whose jobs involve a lot of physical activity also have high H.D.L. levels.

For those non-diabetics who decide to take up regular exercise, the findings of the different studies reported do vary but some studies show a reduction in harmful blood fat particles. The results of the studies are to some extent affected by the amount of physical exercise performed, as a large amount of exercise is necessary to achieve a reduction in levels of blood fats.

There is less information available about the effects of regular physical exercise on blood fats in diabetics. However, a study on the subject was published about twenty years ago in the *Lancet*, by a group of research workers from the famous Karolinska Institute in Stockholm, Sweden. They performed a series of experiments on young people with diabetes, noting the effects of different types of exercise on blood fats. One of these studies involved regular physical activity over a 5-month period consisting of gymnastics, skiing, swimming and running. It is interesting that the levels of blood fat particles tended to fall during this period. It could be due to improved diabetic control, or to an effect of the exercise programme unrelated to control.

In a more recent study this matter was examined closely. Increases in the levels of H.D.L. particles were found in volunteers with diabetes, following an exercise programme, which seemed to be additional to that due to improved diabetic control. More information is required on the effects of exercise on blood fats but, from the studies done in non-diabetics, it is very likely that blood fat levels should show an improvement in response to regular exercise in people with diabetes. However, it seems that the level of activity necessary to see this improvement is quite high and only the keenest sportsmen are likely to see marked changes for the better in terms of their blood fat levels. Moderate exercise is certainly not detrimental and in the well controlled person blood fat levels may even fall.

PHYSICAL FITNESS

Those of you who have a fairly sedentary life without regular exercise are probably 'unfit'. The description 'unfit' does not mean that there is anything wrong with your heart, lungs, alimentary system or any other organ for that matter. What it does mean is that your body as a machine, particularly its muscles, heart and circulation, cannot perform as efficiently as it might.

You may be quite capable of running a short distance to catch the bus or train, or push-starting a car on a cold morning – even untrained and unfit muscles can, in fact, respond to short bursts of heavy physical activity. They are able to do this through a mechanism called anaerobic metabolism. This process can produce energy for muscle work without the need for additional oxygen, as muscle cells store a small amount of oxygen in a pigment similar to the haemoglobin of blood called myoglobin. This oxygen allows the breakdown of glucose to lactate with the release of energy but, after about a minute or so, the muscles switch to aerobic metabolism which requires more oxygen. It is this form of metabolism which is undeveloped and inefficient in the untrained person. So 'unfit' people may be able to perform short bursts of activity (anaerobic metabolism) relatively well but will notice problems if they try longer periods of exertion. The important difference between the terms 'fit' and 'unfit' rests in the capacity for aerobic metabolism to provide the energy for the working muscles. In the physically fit person there are dramatic changes in the biochemistry of the muscle cells together with important adaptations of the cardiovascular system.

Regular physical activity enables the muscle fibres to take up the necessary oxygen for aerobic metabolism much more efficiently. This is because the very small blood vessels (capillaries) in the muscle can increase in number by over 50 per cent. You will remember that the capillaries are where oxygen diffuses from the blood into the tissues, and carbon dioxide diffuses in the opposite direction. So the increased capillary network in muscle makes oxygen diffusion into the fibres more efficient, and allows a considerable increase in blood flow.

As well as these changes in the capillary blood supply, there are important changes with regard to certain muscle enzymes. Enzymes are the body's catalysts and speed up chemical reactions in the tissues. Important enzymes involved in the use and the production of energy are found in mitochondria – microscopic structures in the muscle fibre. Mitochrondria enlarge and multiply in healthy muscle, so that the activity of the enzymes increases dramatically after physical training.

Trained muscle uses fat, in the form of free fatty acids, as fuel probably because the uptake of these substances is easier due to the large increase in the capillary network. Enzymes needed to transfer the fatty acids to where they are broken down for energy within the cell are increased, as are the enzymes needed to break down the fats. Therefore, the muscle of the unfit person tends to break down carbohydrate and little fat, whereas trained muscle tends to use fat rather than glucose.

You will remember that lactate is produced when glucose is broken down for energy. This process, can make the inside of the muscle cell more acid and this limits the capacity of the cell for further activity. It is likely that the accumulation of lactic acid and consequent changes in the acidity of the cell produces the muscle pain experienced by the unfit person taking unaccustomed exercise.

The major benefit of these important muscle changes to the

physically fit person is that the capacity for physical work increases. Scientists measure this by determining the highest rate at which oxygen can be used for producing muscle energy. It is called the maximum oxygen uptake per minute. This measure of fitness can increase by as much as 100 per cent after 8 to 12 weeks training. A person's endurance for physical activity will increase and any given amount of exercise will represent a smaller percentage of that individual's maximum capacity. In simple terms, the person can perform the activity with much less effort than he used at the start.

Physical training also has important effects on the heart and circulation. First of all, because muscle is much more efficient at removing oxygen and fuel substances from the blood, there is less need for an increase in the output of the heart. For any given activity the muscle blood flow will be lower in the fit than in the unfit person. This means that the blood flow to other parts of the body is not reduced as much and consequently the physiological function of these organs is not adversely affected.

Training has a marked effect on the heart itself and for a given level of physical work the heart rate is lower in the trained compared with the untrained person. In addition, the resting heart rate is lower but there is little difference in the maximum heart rate between the trained and untrained. The importance of these changes in heart rate lies in the amount of work that the heart muscle or myocardium has to perform for a given amount of exercise.

Heart rate along with the pressure in the arteries and the amount of blood pumped from the heart in one beat (the stroke volume) determine the amount of energy used by the heart muscle. Therefore, if the heart rate is slower in the physically fit the amount of work necessary by the heart during exercise is reduced. Of course, if the heart rate is slower and the amount of blood being pumped by the heart (cardiac output) stays the same, it means that more blood is pumped by each beat of the heart. The stroke volume of the heart is closely linked with measures of physical fitness. The importance of physical training on the heart is that the cardiac output is higher for any given pulse rate because the amount of blood pumped at each beat is increased and during very heavy exercise, when the heart is beating at its maximum rate, its output will be higher in the trained person, therefore permitting greater amounts of exercise.

It is important to remember that these changes in muscle biochemistry and the heart and circulation do not develop overnight, and physical fitness cannot be obtained instantly. The changes begin to develop in response to increased activity over a longer period, say about eight weeks. The amount of activity is important too. There should be at least 4 periods of exercise during the week and each period should last about half an hour. The amount of exercise should be fairly strenuous. Using the measure of fitness described, i.e., the maximum oxygen uptake per minute, the activity should reach about 70 per cent of this maximum. Such exercise would certainly make you sweat and pant. To give you some idea, imagine riding a bicycle up a fairly steep hill for half an hour. This is the sort of exercise required. Your heart rate will more than double.

Another important point to note is that the beneficial changes in the heart and muscles only remain if the training continues. If activity stops, then the heart and muscle slowly revert to the untrained state, usually over the same sort of time period that they took to improve. Therefore, if you have an enforced lay off from regular activity, then it is necessary to build up the activity again slowly.

8

EXERCISE IN THE OLDER PERSON ON INSULIN

Around the age of 35 most people tend to become less active. It is the age when people may give up their regular sporting activities. This means that the consumption of calories in exercise will be less and if the diet stays the same then the weight will start to increase, and being overweight is not a good idea for the person with diabetes just as for the non-diabetic.

On the other hand, perhaps you are in your 30s and have never really been used to any sort of exercise or sport. Perhaps when you were a child attitudes were different and because of your diabetes you were advised not to take up sport. In the past, of course, it was more difficult to cope with exercise and sport because, for instance, there was no home monitoring of blood glucose. It is not too late to start taking regular exercise and to reap the benefits of physical fitness.

For the older diabetic there are additional problems to be overcome as well as the problems of hypoglycaemia. A youngster can suddenly decide to play football or go on a cross-country run and generally manage quite easily. This is not the case for the older person, whether diabetes is present or not. I am sure that you will have read of middle-aged people joining the jogging craze or suddenly taking up a very active game, such as squash, and having diastrous results. Some people have collapsed with heart attacks after starting to take part in activities far beyond their ability in terms of their own physical fitness. Common sense should suggest that for the older person it is unwise suddenly to take up a high degree of physical activity. For this reason I have devoted a section to general advice on starting exercise and sport specifically for the older diabetic.

In addition to the problems related to being physically unfit, the older person with diabetes will usually have had the condition for longer and various complications may have begun to develop. These can affect the individual's ability to take part in various activities and must be taken into account. However, in most cases some form of physical activity is possible.

PROBLEMS WHICH MAY ARISE

Most people with diabetes live a full, healthy life and the benefits of regular exercise detailed throughout the book certainly contribute to this, along with intelligent use of diet and insulin. There is more and more scientific evidence to suggest that using these three basic components of therapy, to achieve good diabetic control, substantially reduces the possibility of long-term problems. For this reason a lot of effort is given by doctors and people with diabetes for the achievement of good control. This goal has been made less difficult with the introduction of home monitoring of blood glucose levels, multiple insulin injections and measurement of glycosylated haemoglobin, which gives a good overall measure of diabetic control. However, some people do develop complications after many years of diabetes.

The effects of diabetic complications may influence the sort of exercise and sport that is possible. After many years of diabetes, particularly if the control has not been as good as it might, the very small blood vessels known as capillaries may be damaged. These become thicker but more leaky and sometimes are completely blocked. This problem shows itself especially in the eyes and in the kidneys and may also contribute to nerve damage.

Kidneys
The two kidneys are responsible for filtering the blood plasma and removing waste products of the body's metabolism into the urine. They regulate the salt and water content of the blood and reabsorb and conserve the useful components of the blood plasma. The main filtering unit of the kidney is called the glomerulus and there are about a million of these in each kidney. Each glomerulus is full of capillaries so any diabetic capillary damage will affect the function of these vitally important structures.

Because of the importance of kidneys for the disposal of waste products, they receive a very high proportion of the blood pumped by the heart (about a quarter) and it is a very interesting finding that in the early stages of diabetes this flow can increase still further. Whether the increased flow has any adverse effects on the kidney is, as yet, unknown. In the long term, particularly following unsatisfactory diabetic control, the glomerular capillaries may become damaged and leaky. This is detected by the presence of the protein albumin in the urine. Later on the glomeruli become blocked and the ability of these structures to filter the waste products of the blood is reduced and the kidney functions less well. It is to be expected that the problem will decline in the future as emphasis is placed on good diabetic control. It is interesting to note that the very early stages of diabetic kidney damage, when the amount of protein lost in the urine is very small and can only be detected by sophisticated measuring techniques, can be reversed by improving control.

If as sometimes happens, long-term diabetes leads to severe kidney impairment, then it is treated just as it is in non-diabetics by the kidney machine (dialysis) and kidney transplantation. I am sure you will have read that the success of this treatment has improved significantly in recent years.

Exercise may increase the amount of protein found in the urine of diabetic people who have kidney impairment. However, I do not think that anybody knows whether this is important or not. I believe that if you have kidney impairment your ability to take part in exercise and sporting activities will be influenced more by the other factors I have discussed.

Eyes

Damage to the eyes is more likely to occur if control over the years has not been satisfactory. The vision can be affected in several ways. The retina, which is the light-sensitive tissue at the back of the eye, contains a large number of blood capillaries and these capillaries can be damaged by diabetes. This can actually be seen at a very early stage by a doctor using a special instrument called an ophthalmoscope. Damage to the walls of the capillaries can be seen as small red dots known as microaneurysms. These microaneurysms can leak blood which appears as small haemorrhages in the retina.

The capillaries may also become blocked, causing poor blood supply to the retina and consequent damage to its normal function. This process seems to stimulate the growth of new abnormal capillaries which are very friable and tend to bleed. It can be serious as bleeding can occur into the vitreous jelly of the eye and cloud vision. Detachment of the retina can also occur.

I have described the changes in the back of the eye which can occur after many years of diabetes. This may affect the advisability of active sport and exercise and again needs careful discussion with the clinic doctor and also the eye surgeon. Most people accept that it is sensible to avoid strenuous activities if there are abnormal new blood vessels at the back of the eye (proliferative retinopathy). These activities can increase the pressure within the eye and it is likely that the increased pressure could lead to rupture of the blood vessels and bleeding into the vitreous jelly. If you have retinopathy or have had treatment for retinopathy please talk to your doctor before starting an exercise programme.

Fortunately, in recent years a successful treatment has been developed for the early stages of this condition which can prevent further deterioration of vision. The treatment involves the use of a laser beam of light applied to the affected areas of the retina. For the condition to be detected at an early stage, it is necessary for the person with diabetes to have his or her eyes examined at least once a year. Sometimes leaky capillaries around the most sensitive area of the retina cause a condition known as macula oedema, which can result in blurred vision. This can again be treated with the laser beam.

Nerves

When their diabetes is first diagnosed most people notice some abnormal sensations in their arms or legs. These may be aching feelings, numbness or common 'pins and needles'. As the blood glucose is brought under control by insulin treatment these abnormal sensations quickly disappear. Presumably, the uncontrolled diabetic state alters the metabolism of the nerves and it settles down once the diabetes is treated.

After many years of diabetes, and especially if the diabetes has not been well controlled, longstanding damage to nerves can occur. The condition (neuropathy) particularly affects the nerves which carry sensations from the feet and legs and, if severe, can result in loss of normal sensation. If the sensation of pain is lost then knowledge of any injury to the foot is absent. The chapter on foot care is doubly important in this situation and particular care is needed if exercise or sport is undertaken; also, detailed discussion with the chiropodist in the clinic is well worthwhile. Occasionally, along with the damage to nerves affecting the feet, there is poor circulation to the feet and legs. This can show itself as pain in the muscles of the legs which comes on with exercise and goes away at rest. Doctors call the pain intermittent claudication. People with intermittent claudication are encouraged to use their legs as much as possible, as it helps new blood vessels to form in the legs which improves the blood supply. So in this situation meticulous care of the feet is required.

Diabetes can also affect the nerves in the body which generally control those body functions which take place automatically. Damage to these nerves can affect the ability of the body to maintain a normal response to exercise. Also the nerves supplying pain sensation to the heart can be lost, leading to inability to detect the warning chest pain when the heart oxygen supply is limited by coronary heart disease.

For all these reasons the person with diabetes over the age of thirty-five, or who has had diabetes for a long time, should take additional care with sport and exercise. If you come into this older group of people taking insulin and wish to start some form of sporting or exercise programme or wish to continue with your youthful sporting pastimes well into middle age, I can illustrate some of the important points which you will wish to discuss with your doctor.

I have explained about the possibility of disease in the arteries beginning to develop in middle life. This normally shows itself by the symptom called angina. It is a very severe pain across the middle of the chest which comes on during exercise and tends to go away on resting. Sometimes the pain is also felt down the arm and up into the neck. The pain is a warning sign that the heart muscle is not receiving enough oxygen to enable it to pump the extra blood needed for exercise. There are very effective medical and surgical measures available for this condition.

Angina can develop in the middle-aged longstanding diabetic person, just as in the non-diabetic, and the same medicines can be equally effective for both. It is important to remember that the presence of angina does not necessarily mean that exercise is not possible. In fact, more and more authorities are now advocating exercise programmes for people known to have diseased coronary arteries, even those who have already had a heart attack. A detailed description of these exercise programmes is beyond the scope of this book but in the section on further reading I recommend useful publications on the topic.

Some people who have had diabetes for many years develop damage in the autonomic nerves and sometimes the nerves to and from the heart are involved in this process. The sensations from the heart muscle are carried in these nerve fibres and it is possible that angina pain may not be felt, and so the useful warning sign of poor circulation to the heart muscle is lost. It is important that the situation is identified and a special test called the exercise-electrocardiogram has been developed to test the electrical activity in the heart. This is measured during increasing amounts of exercise on a treadmill. If the heart muscle is short of oxygen during the exercise, it shows as a change in the electrical tracing of the heart. This then enables the assessment of the coronary arteries and their ability to deliver the increased blood needed for exercise.

When autonomic nerve damage is extensive it can affect other processes in the body that are important in the physiological response to exercise. It may affect the ability of the heart to beat at different speeds and also the control of blood pressure. So these factors, together with the possibility of loss of angina pain, need detailed discussion between the older diabetic person and his doctor before starting exercise.

STARTING EXERCISE

From what I have said, you will realise that if you are an older person with diabetes, and unused to physical activity, it would be unadvisable suddenly to attempt a sporting activity. If you would like to improve your physical fitness, however, you should start by walking. In my opinion, and I am sure that many of my colleagues will agree, it is the best exercise to start with. Obviously it is difficult to lay down a schedule that will be suitable for all but I will try to give some general guidelines.

Following years of inactivity muscle and ligaments may become weak and any unaccustomed exertion may lead to torn muscles and aching joints. If this happens it may dampen your enthusiasm. Therefore, be patient and start slowly. A simple plan is to walk a short distance, say about a mile twice a day. An advantage of this form of exercise is that it can usually be quite easily incorporated into the daily routine. For instance, walk to the station instead of catching the bus or take the dog for a walk.

In the beginning it may take you as long as half an hour to walk a mile but you will be surprised at your progress in a few weeks. I would keep to this sort of distance for a couple of weeks but take one day off. After two weeks you will have walked twenty-four miles, by which time you will probably be able to start increasing the distance of each walk. Do not rush it: increase the distance by a small amount, say, a quarter of a mile each week. You will certainly begin to feel fitter by this stage and, as well as increasing the distance walked, you will also be able to speed up the pace at which you walk. The speed of a brisk walking pace is approximately three to four miles per hour, so if you walk at this pace for half an hour twice a day you will be covering three to four miles each day. This amounts to as much as twenty-four miles a week assuming one day's rest – a considerable amount of exercise. Walking briskly the body uses about 300 calories per hour and so helps to keep the weight down and the diabetes controlled.

When you have achieved such a level of activity and can perform it comfortably you can then go one step further and try jogging, swimming or cycling. But again remember to build up slowly. During these activities the body uses approximately twice the amount of calories as brisk walking, that is, about 600 calories per hour. You will obviously have to take care to avoid 'hypos' both during and after exercise and give considerable thought to foot care as described in Chapter 4.

9

SOME DIABETICS' PERSONAL EXPERIENCES

One of the best ways of learning about diabetes is to talk to others with the condition. This is why the local branch meetings, the summer camps and the parent/child weekends organised by the B.D.A. are so helpful to the newly diagnosed. I asked several people who I look after in my clinic to explain how they cope with diabetes and their sporting activities.

P.T., AGED 21 YEARS

Peter's diabetes started when he was nine years old. It developed relatively slowly and by the time the diagnosis was made Peter had probably had diabetes for about 6 months. At the beginning, his symptoms were vague, with some loss of energy but he could still take part in games, which he thoroughly enjoyed. At that time he was keen on swimming, cricket and P.E. lessons. After some 3 months he became more and more thirsty and started to lose weight. These symptoms, together with the fact that he was passing more and more urine, led to his doctor testing (with Clinitest tablets) the urine for glucose and sure enough there was 2 per cent glycosuria. There were no ketones present and admission to hospital was arranged so that Peter could be started on insulin injections. Diabetic liaison nurses now enable some people with diabetes to start insulin therapy at home but in the early 1970s Peter had to be admitted to hospital.

In hospital although his blood glucose was high at 15 mmol/l there was no sign of ketosis. He was started on twice-a-day insulin injections, but the insulin dose had to be decreased because of hypoglycaemia. As little as 4 units of lente insulin taken in the morning produced a 'hypo' late in the afternoon. The doctors looking after Peter stopped the insulin and continued his treatment with the diabetic diet alone. In fact, Peter did not go back on insulin injections for 5 months, when he was started on soluble insulin in a dose of 5 units twice a day. Again, on this dose of insulin Peter had 'hypo' attacks and his doctor cut the insulin down to 3 units twice a day. Later he was changed to a once-a-day injection of a lente insulin.

Peter's dose of insulin gradually increased and 3 years after his diagnosis he was changed to twice daily insulin injections. By this time he needed 40 units of insulin per day given as twice-a-day injections of soluble insulin.

For the past 5 years Peter's diabetes has been controlled by Actrapid and Monotard insulin in the following dose:

	a.m.	p.m.
Actrapid	16	18
Monotard	24	10

This is balanced by the following carbohydrate intake:

Breakfast	Snack	Lunch	Snack	Dinner	Snack
45g	20g	45g	20g	55g	20g

Peter is reading History at university and when not studying he enjoys his sporting activities. In the summer he plays cricket for the college team, on a more casual basis enjoys tennis and windsurfing, and plays squash all year round.

Cricket matches during the season take place on Wednesday and Saturday afternoons. They consist of 30 overs a side but Peter's side usually have an hour's practice in the nets before the start of the match proper. Peter bats at number 6 and is disappointed if he does not make at least 20 or 30 runs. He is equally disappointed if he is not handed the ball by his captain to come on and bowl at medium pace at first change. He makes quite a contribution to the side with his batting and bowling. Incidentally, he also fields in the covers which often necessitates some energetic attempts to prevent the ball reaching the boundary.

On match days Peter has his normal insulin in the morning, together with his normal carbohydrate for breakfast, mid-morning snack and lunch. Nets start at 1.30 p.m. and as Peter generally has to bowl for a full hour at his colleagues in the nets, he has half a large Mars bar (50g carbohydrate; 310 calories) halfway through the session. This extra carbohydrate is enough to prevent him developing a 'hypo' for the rest of the nets and the first innings, but he does keep the other half of the Mars bar in his pocket just in case. Tea is taken around 4.00 p.m. and Peter usually has an extra 20g carbohydrate in the form of a brown bread sandwich. At the end of the match Peter checks his blood glucose level and if this is below 6 mmol/l he eats the rest of the Mars bar.

His tennis games during the summer are not planned in advance but usually depend on the availability of partners and courts. However, early afternoon seems to be the commonest time. Peter's efforts at tennis are energetic but not particularly expert. Because of the pressures of his studies and the time devoted to cricket, his tennis matches are restricted to about an hour during which, depending on how well his game is match-ed to that of his opponent, he plays 3 sets. Peter takes his extra carbohydrate in the form of a twin chocolate bar, Twix (37g carbohydrate; 275 calories). About 15 minutes before the match he eats one piece of the Twix and at the end he eats the other piece. Peter initially had problems with hypoglycaemia during his tennis but finds that the Twix bar does the trick in prevent-ing a 'hypo'. He still checks his blood glucose occasionally before and after his tennis to give himself confidence and I can show you two of his blood glucose profiles. One day he played tennis between 3.00 and 4.00 p.m. taking the Twix bar as I have said. His blood glucose tests were:

2.00 p.m. 10.0 mmol/l
4.30 p.m. 13.3 ,,
6.30 p.m. 6.7 ,,
10.00 p.m. 4.4 ,,

On another day when he played tennis between 2.30 p.m. and 3.30 p.m. his blood tests were:

2.00 p.m. 6.7 mmol/l
4 p.m. 10.0 ,,
7 p.m. 6.7 ,,
10 p.m. 6.7 ,,

Peter's other summer sporting activity is windsurfing. He is fortunate that his college has a windsurfing club which owns six boards together with a suitably adapted minibus to carry the club members and boards to the lake. This activity usually takes place on Sundays and the club set out early and reach the water by mid-morning. He was lucky to be able to learn to windsurf on a specialised two week holiday in the Greek islands. Apparently, when beginning this sport you are in the water more often than actually on the board so it does help if you can learn in a warm climate. Certainly for enjoyable sport in Britain Peter finds his wet-suit essential.

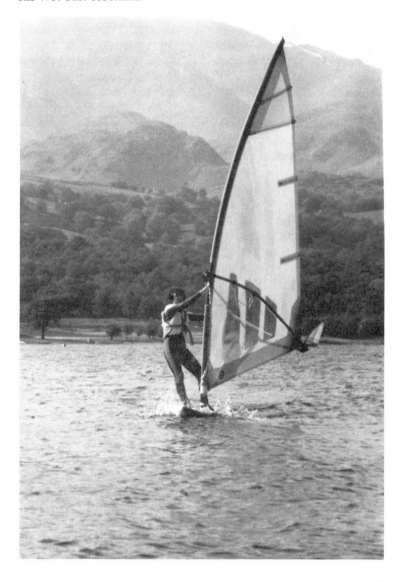

When Peter was learning to windsurf and was continually having to heave himself out of the water back on to the board he found that his additional requirements for carbohydrate were quite high. He also reduced his morning insulin by 20 per cent. He took his extra glucose as a drink of Coke which as well as preventing a 'hypo' kept him hydrated under the hot Greek sun! He needed to drink a can of Coke (135g carbohydrate; 135 calories) for each 2-hour session.

His current way of protecting himself from hypoglycaemia is to reduce his morning insulin by 8 units on windsurfing days, so that he takes 12 units of Actrapid and 20 units of Monotard insulin. He has his usual 20g mid-morning snack before putting his board in the water at about 11.00 a.m. After an hour he stops and drinks half a small bottle of Lucozade. At about 1.00 p.m. he stops with his club-mates for lunch, which usually consists of a picnic washed down by a can of lager. During the afternoon session Peter drinks the rest of the Lucozade at about 3.30 p.m. He has had problems with late hypoglycaemia on Sunday evenings following a day of windsurfing and he takes an extra 20g carbohydrate with his evening meal which seems to prevent this happening.

I must emphasize that windsurfing is a potentially hazardous sport, especially on large expanses of water. Peter never goes windsurfing on his own and he always keeps warm with the wet suit and wears a life jacket. His club mates are aware of his diabetes and know the first aid drill for dealing with a 'hypo'.

G.L., AGED 31 YEARS

Gill is a school physical education teacher. She developed diabetes only a year ago. The onset of her diabetic symptoms was slow and, in fact, she first came to the hospital because of a red mark on her shin. It turned out to be a very rare skin condition occasionally seen in diabetic people, known as necrobiosis lipoidica. A routine test of the urine showed glucose and an appointment was made for the clinic. It was only in the few days before she attended the diabetic clinic that she started to feel thirsty and by that time her blood glucose was 23.4 mmol/l. She was very reluctant to start insulin injections and insisted on trying the effect of diet and tablets first. Her grandmother had diabetes and was well controlled on tablets and Gill hoped the same would be true for her.

Although her glucose level fell a little on tablets she quickly realised that she needed insulin. She had no energy and felt very weak. She soon got used to the insulin injections and discovered that they were not as bad as she had thought. In fact she was very grateful because after a week or two she felt her old self and could turn out for the local hockey team again! Her skin condition has also improved considerably.

Gill has 2 insulin injections each day. She takes a mixture of Humulin S and Humulin Zn in a dose of 4 units of Humulin S and Zn before breakfast, and 2 units of Humulin S and 4 units of Humulin Zn before the evening meal. Gill's insulin dose is quite low which means that her own pancreas is still producing some insulin. Her insulin is balanced against a diet containing 45g carbohydrate for each of her main meals together with 10g snacks.

Gill's main sporting activities outside her duties at school are hockey and skiing in the winter months, and swimming in the summer. She has three to four opportunities of skiing every year as she supervises various school trips. Skiing is heavy exercise, both the cross-country type and the downhill, and care is obviously needed to prevent 'hypos' in skiers with diabetes. This is of additional importance as the weather in the high mountains can be very cold (see Chapter 4). Gill always skis in a group and is well prepared for cold weather by wearing thermal underwear and a thick quilted ski suit. She also carries a space blanket for emergency use.

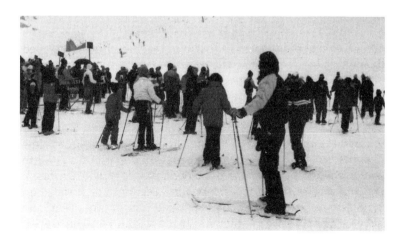

At the beginning of her skiing day Gill takes her usual insulin and breakfast but when she has got to the top of the mountain (about 10.00 a.m.) after the usual long queue for the cable car she takes some additional carbohydrate. She is very fond of chocolate coconut bars and has found that to cope with two hours hard skiing she has to eat a double Bounty (37g carbohydrate; 300 calories). She stops for lunch at about 12 noon and has an extra 20g carbohydrate and then halfway through the afternoon session at about 3.00 p.m. she has a Blue Ribbon chocolate bar (12g carbohydrate; 105 calories). Taking these precautions Gill has not had any diabetic problems when skiing.

Gill turns out for her local hockey team every Saturday afternoon in the winter time. She plays in defence. The hockey matches start at 2.30 p.m. and she has her normal insulin, breakfast and lunch before the match. Just before going on the field she eats a Yorkie chocolate bar (35g carbohydrate; 320 calories) which she finds sufficient to prevent a 'hypo'. When she first started playing hockey again after her diabetes was treated with insulin she checked her blood glucose at half-time and in general the reading was about 7 mmol/l. At half-time she has the usual half orange (5g carbohydrate) with the rest of the team. So far she has not found it necessary to take extra carbohydrate with her evening meal on Saturday to prevent a late 'hypo'.

Swimming is Gill's sporting occupation in the summer months and again she makes use of her favourite chocolate bars. She has no set times for swimming and often she decides on the spur of the moment to visit the swimming baths. For a short session lasting about an hour she finds that a single Bounty bar is sufficient. Sometimes she has a double bar if she is doing some serious training. When she swims in competitions she again has a small chocolate bar. After swimming, especially after a heavy session, she has a can of ordinary Coca Cola.

V.N., AGED 28 YEARS

Vivienne developed diabetes when she was 13 but it has never stood in her way either academically (she will shortly qualify as a medical doctor) or in sport. Because of her duties as a medical student she has found it difficult to keep to set meal times and quickly decided that the best plan for her was to have multiple insulin injections to allow herself more flexibility. Initially, this consisted of 16 units Actrapid insulin before breakfast and before lunch. Then before the evening meal she took 16 units of Actrapid insulin combined with 16 units of Insulatard insulin (pork monocomponent isophane insulin made by Nordisk). However, when she started her work on the wards in the hospital she found that it was difficult to stick to a set time for her evening injection and meal. This led to problems with her diabetic control due to the changing time of injection of the Insulatard. She got over this by splitting the evening injection. She took the Actrapid insulin before her evening meal whenever she managed to have it and then took the Insulatard insulin at bedtime. Recently she has used the Novopen to administer human Actrapid insulin before her meals and finds the method very convenient.

Vivienne is keen on many sports, swims regularly, plays squash and cycles. She also enjoys fell walking and horse riding. Of all these she has found squash the most difficult to cope with from the diabetic point of view but she now manages to enjoy the sport along with her other activities. Her main problem with squash was 'hypo' attacks. These started fairly early in the match. Usually, having won the first game easily, sometimes without her opponent scoring a point, she would 'go to pieces' and lose the next game as easily as she had won the first. She now manages to play at her best throughout a rigorous 45-minute squash game (squash is very demanding in terms of energy expenditure and the body uses over 10 kilocalories each minute).

The most important factor in Vivienne's experience to ensure trouble-free squash has been the timing of the game. She discovered that 6.00 p.m. was the best time. This is probably because the effective insulin activity in her body before her evening injection will be quite low. You will remember that a particular problem with diabetes and sport is that the injected insulin will continue being absorbed into the blood even though the body's requirement for insulin in this situation is low.

Before the squash match Vivienne takes extra carbohydrate and enjoys a two-finger Kit Kat (14g carbohydrate; 115 calories). She finds this is sufficient to maintain her glucose level for the game. Vivienne has not had any problems with later 'hypos' and does not take extra carbohydrate with her evening meal after squash.

Vivienne's other sporting and outdoor activities have not

created the same difficulties as the squash. She takes a 90-minute swimming session in her stride after an extra 30g carbohydrate in the form of chocolate biscuits. For fell or mountain walks she starts the day with an extra 20g carbohydrate for breakfast and she sometimes reduces her morning Actrapid insulin by 4 units as well. During the walk she maintains her glucose level with a couple of Dextrosol tablets. She always knows when to take extra glucose. I have now actually persuaded her to check her blood glucose level at intervals; she does not find this too inconvenient and her Autolet and testing strips fit easily into a pocket of her pack. I should emphasize that Vivienne is a very sensible person and does not underestimate the potential hazards of the fells and mountains. She never goes alone and is well prepared for rapid changes in weather conditions.

Vivienne is also a keen cyclist and, in fact, uses her cycle for regular commuting to London. For these relatively short rides she does not need to take extra carbohydrate. However, on cycling holidays when she may cycle for 2–3 hours at a time she adopts a similar regime to that for her fell walking. If the afternoon is going to be as tough as the morning she also has an extra 20g carbohydrate for lunch and again takes 4 units less of her Actrapid insulin.

Horse riding seems to require much less in the way of extra glucose, and when Vivienne is hacking out at a fairly leisurely pace she tends not to take any extra. The energy expended when she is schooling horses requires more exertion and before a session she will take a two-finger Kit Kat.

I.P., AGED 16

Ian developed diabetes less than 2 years ago. He became ill over a few days with a severe thirst and passed large quantities of urine. His weight fell by half a stone and he felt very weak indeed. He was ill enough to be admitted to hospital but was home again after a few days. Ian was quick to understand the basics of diabetes and was stabilised with two injections a day of Actrapid and Monotard insulin. He was rather reluctant to start home monitoring of his blood glucose but now finds it a tremendous advantage. From the beginning Ian has injected into his abdomen.

Ian has always enjoyed sport, particularly swimming and badminton, and was upset at the outset of his diabetes because he felt he would not be able to participate again. I reassured him but he believed me only when he felt stronger and started to put on weight again with the insulin injections.

It is interesting to see how Ian has coped with his sporting activities, as he has experience with two different insulin regimes. Previously, Ian's insulin dosage was:

	a.m.	*p.m.*
Actrapid	7	9
Monotard	14	8

Instead of taking both insulins before the evening meal he had the Actrapid and then the Monotard at bedtime. Splitting the evening injection in this way gave Ian more flexibility in how he spent his evening and what time he had his meal.

Games afternoon at Ian's school is on Wednesday, and his afternoon starts with a swimming session between 2.30 and 3.45 p.m. Ian practises all his strokes and occasionally races are organised. The amount of energy expended by swimming varies a little on the actual stroke – breast and back stroke, for instance, are classified as heavy work using between 7.5 and 9 kilocalories per minute, whereas the crawl stroke is heavy work using more than 10 kilocalories per minute. After the swimming session Ian plays badminton from 4.00 to 5.00 p.m. Badminton, depending on the intensity with which the game is played, ranges between moderate and heavy work. Ian finds badminton more strenuous than his swimming but this may be due to the order in which he does them.

Until the start of his sporting afternoon Ian keeps his diabetic day unaltered. Possible approaches would have been to take a reduction in the morning dose of Monotard insulin and/or to take extra carbohydrate exchanges for the Wednesday midday meal. However, Ian was reluctant to change his insulin for the day and found that swimming after extra bulky carbohydrates was uncomfortable. He found that Dextrosol tablets provided him with the extra glucose he required. He took two tablets before starting to swim and then a further four tablets at intervals during the swimming. Before badminton he took another two Dextrosol and during the game a further two. This additional quick acting glucose enables Ian to play his two sports competitively. To begin with Ian tended to have 'hypos' in the early hours (about 1.00 a.m.) of Thursday morning. He has resolved the problem by taking an extra 20g carbohydrate with his evening meal.

In recent months Ian's insulin regime has changed. He was quite keen on trying the injection device called Novopen, which makes injections more convenient. The instrument is very similar, as its name suggests, to a pen (see photo on page 10). Inside there is a cartridge (a Penfill) of human Actrapid insulin. When the cap of the 'pen' is removed a fine needle (disposable) is revealed and a window in the barrel of the pen shows the contents of the insulin cartridge. The cap screws on to the end of the pen and forms the plunger of the pen syringe. Each full press of this plunger (it makes a clicking sound) delivers two units of insulin. The Novopen has really been designed to help in the giving of mulitiple injections each day, and human Actrapid is given before breakfast and the evening meal. A basal insulin supplement is given at bedtime as Human Ultratard, a very long acting insulin. The idea is to separate the basal insulin requirement (Ultratard) from the insulin needed to cover meals (Actrapid). It allows a lot of flexibility, particularly with the timing of meals. As the Novopen is portable it makes it easier to give an injection before the midday meal. On this regime the extra injection is usually necessary unless a very light lunch and no afternoon snack are taken.

When Ian first used the pen he was reluctant to reduce his lunch, as he gets very hungry in the middle of the day. Ian took 18 units of human Ultratard at bedtime (this injection is given in the usual way) and human Actrapid with the Novopen before breakfast (10 units) and before the evening meal (8 units). His blood glucose tests at home averaged about 6 mmol/l, apart from before his evening meal when they were high at 13 mmol/l. It was obvious that he needed an injection before his lunch and he now takes 6 units of human Actrapid at this time.

Ian copes with Wednesday afternoon sports in a different way. He finds that by omitting his lunchtime Actrapid injection he can get through his swimming and badminton sessions without so many Dextrosol tablets. He takes two Dextrosol before swimming and two before badminton. He still finds it necessary to take an extra 20g carbohydrate with his evening meal.

M.P., AGED 64

Margaret developed the classical symptoms of diabetes 30 years ago at the age of 34 and has been on insulin injections since then. It is of interest that her mother also had insulin dependent diabetes but she did not develop her diabetes until the age of 82 years. Despite 30 years of diabetes Margaret has no evidence of diabetic problems, which she attributes to good diabetic control and a very active lifestyle.

Until she retired at the age of 60 years she worked as a superintendent physiotherapist and had to be physically fit to cope with the demands of rehabilitating patients in the gymnasium. Since her retirement Margaret has stayed very active indeed. She loves foreign travel and is always going to various remote corners of the world. Since she started measuring blood glucose rather than testing urine, she finds that her diabetes is much easier to handle on these trips, which often involve long flights. She uses the Visidex blood testing strips and pricks her finger with the Autolet machine.

Her current insulin regime consists of twice daily injections of Humulin I and Humulin S. Before breakfast she takes 12 units of Humulin S and 8 units of Humulin I, and before dinner she takes 3 units of Humulin S and 8 units of Humulin I. This is balanced against a carbohydrate intake as follows:

Breakfast	Snack	Lunch	Snack	Dinner	Snack
55g	20g	45g	20g	55g	20g

At the age of 64, Margaret does not take part in sport in the true sense but she is involved in activities requiring physical exertion such as gardening and birdwatching. She has quite a big garden and manages all the work herself. Some of the gardening chores, such as digging, are very energetic indeed. Mowing the lawn and general gardening jobs such as weeding involve moderate work. In the past Margaret has certainly provoked 'hypos' with her gardening activities both at the time and later in the evening. These 'hypos' are now avoided by taking extra carbohydrate. For a particularly heavy session of gardening Margaret takes an extra 20g carbohydrate as digestive biscuits or a wholemeal bread sandwich. She does not seem to need to take extra carbohydrate with her evening meal to prevent delayed 'hypos'.

Margaret's local birdwatching club tends to organise day trips to interesting areas by coach and on most occasions a considerable amount of walking is involved. This certainly requires additional carbohydrate intake. The amount Margaret needs to take obviously depends on the length and the nature of the walk but as a general guideline she uses an extra 10g carbohydrate for each hour of the walk. She may increase this to 20g if the walk is particularly arduous. She has suffered from late 'hypos' after long birdwatching trips and an extra 20g carbohydrate is required for her evening meal. If the trip is going to be especially hard, she occasionally reduces her morning Humulin I insulin from 8 units to 4 units.

M.V., AGED 15

Manuel was 13 when he developed classic diabetic symptoms. He was lucky in that the symptoms were not very severe and he did not become ketotic but he did lose eight pounds in weight. From the beginning Manuel has been treated with twice daily injections of Velosulin (a quick acting pork soluble insulin made by Nordisk) and Insulatard (a pork isophane insulin also from Nordisk) and his current dosage is as follows:

	a.m.	p.m.
Velosulin	12	12
Insulatard	18	10

This insulin is balanced against a daily intake of 230g carbohydrate divided between 3 main meals and 3 snacks. Manuel does measure his blood glucose levels at home but is certainly not London's keenest home monitor! Fortunately, Manuel's diabetes is very stable and his glycosylated haemoglobin level is always normal.

Sport certainly takes a prominent part in Manuel's life. He is an enthusiast for tennis in the summer, plays squash and swims throughout the year. He swims every day after school at 5.00 p.m. and at the weekend. He enjoys diving and spends a quarter of an hour using the spring board and then he generally swims eight lengths of the fifty metre pool. Perhaps because this side of Manuel's sporting activity is so regular and has become part of his normal day he does not seem to require extra carbohydrate before the swim. However, he does have a large (30g) mid-afternoon snack at 3.30 p.m. and after the swimming session he eats a small bag of potato crisps (32g carbohydrate;

245 calories) to avoid the mild 'hypo' symptoms he used to experience before his evening meal.

During the winter Manuel plays squash two days each week at 10.00 a.m. He always books a double session, playing an hour and a half instead of the usual forty-five minutes. Manuel has found two equally effective ways to cope with his squash. He has his usual insulin and breakfast on squash days but before the match he either has a quarter of a large Mars bar or a quarter of a small bottle of Lucozade. During the match he has the rest of the Mars bar or the rest of the Lucozade.

In the summer months Manuel plays tennis during his school games period on Tuesday afternoons. The tennis starts around 2.00 p.m. and lasts for two hours and he takes an extra 20g carbohydrate for his lunch on these days. Manuel finds that the gentler pace of tennis does not require the fast acting glucose supplement that he needs before squash. Halfway through the game he has one or two Dextrasol tablets depending on the speed of the game and he eats a small bag of potato crisps on his way home.

B.S., AGED 8

Ben developed diabetes at the age of 7 years. He became ill over a few days, his main symptoms being drowsiness, fever and a cough. There were no obvious diabetic symptoms and, in fact, diabetes was not suspected at first. However, on routine testing of the urine glucose and ketones were discovered, which made diabetes highly likely, and later his blood glucose was found to be 34.7 mmol/l which confirmed the diagnosis. His blood was quite acid, too, with all the ketones and he needed a drip feed and insulin into a vein to correct this.

Ben's diabetes came as a great shock to him and to his mother but they coped well and Ben quickly felt better. He now has two insulin injections a day, with 14 units of Monotard insulin before breakfast and 4 units before the evening meal. He also has 3 units of Actrapid insulin in the evening but none in the morning. Ben's insulin dose is balanced against a diet of 160g carbohydrate which he divides in the following way:

Breakfast	Snack	Lunch	Snack	Dinner	Snack
30g	20g	50g	10g	40g	10g

Ben's mother helps him with blood glucose tests at home and he is learning to draw up and give the insulin already. Ben prefers the Autolance finger pricking machine because it is almost painless and he uses B.M. strips for blood glucose measurements. Ben's mother is a teacher and she has made sure that his teachers know about Ben's diabetes and how to help him if a 'hypo' occurs. The diabetic liaison sister has also visited the school to see Ben and his teacher.

Ben's elder brother is very good at games and Ben is keen to try to keep up with him. He has a P.E. lesson every morning at about 10.30 during school term. To prevent a 'hypo' during the period which lasts about 40 minutes Ben has a mini crunch bar (15g carbohydrate; 160 calories). He also takes a crunch bar before swimming lessons in the afternoons which last for about 20 minutes. Until he is a little older the liaison sister has asked his teacher to help him remember to eat the crunch bar before P.E. and swimming, and Ben has no problems with hypoglycaemia.

SUGGESTED FURTHER READING

Diabetes: A practical guide for patients on insulin, Robert Tattersall (Churchill Livingstone Patient Handbook 9).

Diabetes: A practical new guide to healthy living, James W. Anderson (Martin Dunitz).

Insulin Dependent Diabetes, John L. Day (Thorsons Publishing Group).

Fit to Exercise, Edmund J. Burke and John H. L. Humphreys (Pelham Books).

Diabetics Guide to Health and Fitness, Kris E. Berg (Eddington Hook Limited).

The Diabetic's Diet Book, Dr Jim Mann (Martin Dunitz).

Diabetes Explained, Dr Arnold Bloom (MTP Press Ltd).

SOME USEFUL ADDRESSES

Ames Division
Miles Laboratories Ltd
P.O. Box 37
Stoke Court
Slough SL24 4LY
(for Glucometer blood glucose machine and Visidex and Glucostix testing strips)

Boehringer Corp (London) Ltd
Bell Lane
Lewes
East Sussex BN7 1LG
(for Reflolux blood glucose machine and BM test 1–44 blood testing strips)

British Diabetic Association
10 Queen Anne Street
London W1

Hypoguard (UK) Ltd
Dock Lane
Melton
Woodbridge
Suffolk IP12 IPE
(for Hypocount blood glucose machine and GA testing strips; many other products can also be obtained from Hypoguard, including the BD Autolance and the Autoclix finger pricking machines)

Medistron Ltd
6 Lawson Hunt Industrial Park
Broadbridge Heath
Horsham
East Sussex RH12 3JR
(for Glucocheck blood glucose machine)

Owen Mumford Ltd
Medical Shop
Brook Hill
Woodstock
Oxon OX7 1BR
(a wide range of self care products including the Autolet finger pricking machinery)

The Sports Council
Information Centre
16 Upper Woburn Place
London WC1H 0QP

The Physical Education
Association
Ling House
162 King's Cross Road
London WC1X 9DH

INDEX

alcohol 58
athlete's foot 58

blood glucose level 27, 49
blood glucose measurement 33
blood pressure 20
body metabolism 17
breathing 19

carbohydrate 9; intake 42
carbon dioxide 18, 22
cholesterol 83
circulation 19

diet 12, 42

energy expenditure of various activities 44
exchanges (carbohydrate) 12
exercise 26; starting 94
eyes 91

fitness 85
footcare 55
footwear 54

glucagon 32
glycogen 23
glyconeogenesis 25
glycosuria 9

haemoglobin 19
heart 19
heat 21
home monitoring 33

hypoglycaemia 13
hypoglycaemia symptoms 29

insulin
    action on metabolism 8
    dosage 47
    injection sites 37
    types of 9

ketoacidosis 14
ketones 9
kidneys 90

lungs 18

muscle metabolism 23

nerves 92
Novopen 10, 106

obesity 80
oxygen 18

pancreas 8
physical training 86
pulse 20

renal threshold for glucose 33

school pack 15
smoking 39
summer camps (B.D.A.) 64; junior 67; teenage 69
sweating 22

weight tables 82